MIDLIFE AWAKENING

ALSO BY MARIANNE WILLIAMSON

A Course in Weight Loss

A Return to Love

A Woman's Worth

Illuminata

Emma & Mommy Talk to God

Healing the Soul of America

Enchanted Love

Everyday Grace

The Gift of Change

Illuminated Prayers

The Law of Divine Compensation

*Miracle Cards**

The Mystic Jesus

A Politics of Love

Tears to Triumph

*A Year of Daily Wisdom Perpetual Flip Calendar**

A Year of Miracles

*Available from Hay House
Please visit:

Hay House USA: www.hayhouse.com®
Hay House Australia: www.hayhouse.com.au
Hay House UK: www.hayhouse.co.uk
Hay House India: www.hayhouse.co.in

MIDLIFE AWAKENING

Creating a Miraculous Next Chapter

MARIANNE WILLIAMSON

HAY HOUSE

HAY HOUSE LLC
Carlsbad, California • New York City
London • Sydney • New Delhi

Published in the United States by: Hay House LLC, www.hayhouse.com® • P.O. Box 5100, Carlsbad, CA, 92018-5100

Cover design: Julie Davison • *Interior design:* Bryn Starr Best

Library of Congress Cataloging-in-Publication Data for the original edition

Williamson, Marianne.
The age of miracles : embracing the new midlife / Marianne Williamson.—1st ed.
p. cm.
ISBN 978-1-4019-1719-7 (hardcover) • ISBN 978-1-4019-1720-3 (tradepaper)
1. Middle age--Psychological aspects.
2. Middle-aged persons--Conduct of life. I. Title.
HQ1059.4.W57 2008
155.6'6--dc22 2007034606

This book was previously published with the title *The Age of Miracles* and the ISBN: 978-1-4019-1720-3

Tradepaper ISBN: 979-8-3186-0157-6
E-book ISBN: 979-8-3186-0158-3
Audiobook ISBN: 979-8-3186-0215-3

10 9 8 7 6 5 4 3 2 1
1st edition, January 2008
2nd edition, October 2025

Printed in the United States of America

This product uses responsibly sourced papers, including recycled materials and materials from other controlled sources.

The authorized representative in the EU for product safety and compliance is Penguin Random House Ireland, Morrison Chambers, 32 Nassau Street, Dublin D02 YH68, Ireland. https://eu-contact.penguin.ie

To India More Nisbett
for the woman you've become

CONTENTS

Preface to the 2025 Edition.................................ix

Introduction xi

CHAPTER 1: The Long and Winding Road 1

CHAPTER 2: Do You Believe in Magic? 11

CHAPTER 3: The Nick of Time 39

CHAPTER 4: God Only Knows 57

CHAPTER 5: Women of a Certain Age 79

CHAPTER 6: I Will Survive 99

CHAPTER 7: In the Midnight Hour 123

CHAPTER 8: Abraham, Martin, and John 139

CHAPTER 9: We Are the World 155

Acknowledgments...171

About the Author..173

[T]horoughly unprepared we take the step
into the afternoon of life;
worse still, we take this step with the false assumption
that our truths and ideals will serve us as hitherto.
But we cannot live the afternoon of life
according to the programme of life's morning;
for what was great in the morning
will be little at evening,
and what in the morning was true
will at evening have become a lie.

— Carl Jung, Stages of Life

Preface
to the 2025 Edition

I published *The Age of Miracles: Embracing the New Midlife* in 2008. Having reached a time in my life when I was about to embark on Chapter 3, I thought I knew what was about to hit me. But of course I didn't. What I wrote at that time, while it told much of the story, couldn't possibly reflect some things I would only learn later.

The process of aging is more mysterious, and more uncharted in its spiritual and emotional aspects, than I had realized. Much was about to unfold in life that surprised me, and I think surprises everyone as they reach the middle years. It reminds me of old-fashioned movies where pioneers ride into territory that very few have ever seen. Pioneers are usually looking not only for a new place to see, but for a new way to be. Midlife today is a space that is new and unmapped that way. It's prime material for reinvention of self.

Reading *The Age of Miracles* again after almost 20 years, I thought to myself, *Oh Lord. This thing is outdated.* A lot has happened in the world since 2008, and many references that made sense then now seemed like old news. Originally thinking we would simply update some excerpts, I was almost mystically paired with an editor who felt, as I did, that the book needed more than that. It needed something more than just a facelift, which ironically is very much the point of the book!

I'm grateful to both Reid Tracy and Anne Barthel for giving me the opportunity to rewrite the material. These are not just words on a page to me, and I hope they won't be for the reader either. May everyone who reads it feel immersed in fine wine.

Marianne Williamson
London

Introduction

Wrinkles. Memory gaps. Can't remember what you did yesterday. Found your glasses in the refrigerator. The skin on your thighs is uneven. Your butt is too soft. Younger people call you "ma'am" (or "sir"). You used to be able to juggle so many more balls in the air. You don't know that face in the mirror anymore. You're jealous of younger people. You can't believe you didn't appreciate it when you had it. You feel invisible. You haven't a clue who's making music now. You used to be hip, but apparently not anymore. . . .

If any of this sounds familiar, then welcome to the territory. Perhaps you could use a fresh layer of insight to help you navigate some shifting ground.

Every new experience confronts you with a choice, and aging is no exception. How the era of "no longer young" unfolds for you—how you'll inhabit the space of midlife and beyond—is an open question that only you can answer. If you choose the path of least resistance—nonresistance not in a Taoist way but in a lazy way—then gravity will overwhelm you. An undertow will pull you down. You'll grow old with little grace or joy.

But if you claim for yourself another possibility, you'll open the door to something decidedly new. Considering the possibility that there might be another way, you'll make room for a miracle. You'll pave another pathway, build new synapses in your brain, and physically and spiritually welcome new energies that would otherwise not find in you a receptive home.

Millions of us are entering a room we would have liked to avoid yet can avoid no longer. Yet if we take a good look, we realize the room doesn't have to be so bad . . . perhaps it just needs a redesign. And then it will be in many ways a new room.

Midlife is not new territory, obviously, but what *is* new is how many of us are reaching for something outside its culturally prescribed norms. According to Werner Erhard, founder of the *est* organization, we can live our lives either acting out of circumstances or acting out of a vision. And when it comes to age, we can forge a new vision, a new conversation, to take us beyond the limited thought-forms that have defined its parameters for generations. The circumstances are fixed, but our experience of them is not. Every situation is experienced within the context of the conversation surrounding it, both in our heads and in our culture. Out of a new conversation about midlife emerges new hope for those of us who find ourselves there.

When I say hope, do I mean the hope of more years? Not necessarily. Do I mean the hope of more fun, more meaning, more passion, more enlightenment? Absolutely. Hope, when it comes to age, is not just that the years get longer but that they get *better.* Recently I sat next to an aging movie star at a wedding reception. Now in his 80s, he told me with manly conviction that when his time came, he would "go willingly, and get on to the next adventure." He seemed okay with whatever happens next because he is okay with whatever happens, period. He seemed connected to some flow of life that's too real to ever stop, that wouldn't dare shut down at the point of his death.

I saw him half an hour later, dancing like Valentino with a woman 50 years younger than himself. Back at the table, I heard him rail against the government like a resplendent Titan who didn't give a damn if what he said was popular or not. It didn't seem like he had reached the end of his life so much as its peak. And at this peak, he could see that what stretched out before him was just a new piece of land, no less real than the territory behind him.

How would we live were we not afraid of death? How would we live if we felt full permission from ourselves and others to give to life everything we've got? Would midlife be time to shut down, or time to finally get started? Would it be time to give up, or time to claim what we really want? Would it be time to just hang out, or time to stop messing around? If we wish to age on autopilot, as a preprescribed and prepackaged experience, then it's certainly not difficult—the status quo has signposts everywhere. But if we want to create something new for ourselves and those around us, then it's important to recognize how limited and limiting are the thoughts about age that still saturate our culture.

And to realize that we can let them go.

Many of our thoughts about midlife are outdated. They are hand-me-down notions from preceding generations that no longer fit who we are or what we're doing here.

I recently met a woman who was a political icon in the '70s and '80s. When I asked her if she wanted to get back into the political fray, she looked at me and said, "Oh no, I'm 66." She pointed to a table of young women behind us, saying, "Let them take over now."

I looked at her, horrified. The women at the table behind us were *not* the ones I could see steering the world in a more positive direction any time soon, and I knew that in her heart, she couldn't either.

"Them? Are you *crazy?*" I gasped, pointing to the table of younger women behind us, trying unsuccessfully to scan their faces for any sign of seriousness. And as I said that, I saw her eyes light up. Perhaps she just needed someone to give her permission to admit what she was already thinking: She's actually more ready now than ever. *She's* someone who's got what it takes.

As she left the table, she told me, "You're right. Let's talk sometime. I want to do something *radical.*"

One shift in perception was all she had needed. Someone simply doubting the notion that her best days were behind her sent her running from a resigned and timid "It's *their* turn now," to a more emotionally honest "It's *my* turn now!" And in our hearts, many of us feel as she does: that we're finally ready to do something radical! Whatever it is we're here for, we're itching to do it now.

But sometimes you're not sure you know what "it" is. And even if you do, you might secretly fear it's too late. You're caught between the excited feeling that you're ready to begin and the scary thought that you might be past your prime. Yet the weight of God's hand supersedes the weight of your personal history. God works miracles anytime, anywhere, for anyone; the last thing that could slow Him down is the fact that you're older than you used to be.

Time seems, when we're younger, to move so slowly. Then all of a sudden it seems to have gone by so fast. Tragic time delays dot the landscape, from women who didn't realize they wanted children until the choice becomes more physically challenging, to people stuck in careers they hate because for years they didn't have the courage to go for what they really wanted. That's why it's so important that we not buy in to the notion that once we've reached midlife, our options are limited. Life will be, at any point, exactly what we program it to be. Yesterday does not have the power to determine our today. Every situation is a challenge to rise to the occasion—or, to put it more accurately, to allow God to *lift* us to the occasion—and midlife is no exception. God is always ready to turn water into wine.

Whomever it is you were born to be, whatever your soul was coded to accomplish, whatever lessons you were born to learn, now is the time to get serious and get going. The more seriously you take life, the more seriously life will seem to take you. It is your thoughts, and your thoughts alone, that determine what's possible for you now. It's time to proactively reach beyond any predetermined formulas you or anyone else might have for what's "possible" at this time in your life. No matter what did or did not happen in your past, the present remains an endless fount of miraculous opportunities—the law of divine compensation guarantees that. "Endless possibility" is not just an abstraction; it is the coding of the universe, an active force of constant and infinite elasticity. It responds not to your past, but to your present state of mind.

It's not what's happened in your life so far that has the power to determine your future. It's how you interpret what's happened, and learn from what's happened, that sets the course for your probable tomorrows.

Life doesn't always (or even usually) move in a consistently rising arc of progress. By the time we're in our 40s, most of us have stumbled in at least one or two major areas: marriage or divorce, problems with kids, career, finances, addiction, or whatever. But the point of a life journey isn't whether or not we've fallen down; it's whether or not we've learned how to get back up. *Everyone* falls because it's a fallen world. It's who gets up, and how they do it, that determines what happens next.

I have a friend who is a fantastic singer, wowing audiences with her voice for years. She's also gorgeous to look at. Everyone has always said she was destined for stardom. But did she get her big break at 20, 30, or even 40? No, because like many of us, her demons held her back for years. She would miss a big meeting because she was hungover, or say the wrong thing to a record executive because her style was immature. She consistently sabotaged her own success. It wasn't until after her 40th birthday that all the pieces came together, her talent and personality aligned at last. And what she could see once that happened—what everyone around her could see—was that the long and winding journey she had taken only added to the luminosity of her success, once it came.

What do I mean by the "luminosity" of her success? I mean the layers of understanding that went into it: the large and small lessons learned along the way that ultimately affected not only her singing but her way of being in the world, a new essence not only to what she does but to who she is. It wasn't just her voice but her personality that had needed to ripen.

Sometimes you can't lift your legs as high in aerobics class anymore, but you can lift a knowing eyebrow in a way that comes only with years of experience. In a way, that eyebrow is more impressive than the leg lift. That's what maturity offers: a new richness to our personality. An understanding that could only have come, as my father used to say, when we've had to "take the good with the bad."

The new maturity is optimistic—not the unknowing optimism of our youth, when all things seemed possible, but rather a bittersweet-yet-knowing optimism, held to in spite of the fact that we now know certain things are *not* any longer possible. We've lost some things we would rather have not lost, but we've made some gains we didn't even know existed. We've "been there, done that" in enough areas to feel we've achieved some mastery, not so much at this or that, but at living a more responsible life. Once we've accepted that life is not as fabulous in some of the ways we thought it was, we realize it's even more fabulous in ways we could never have known.

It's not that you're deluding yourself, refusing to gracefully accept that your youth is over. You accept the limits of age, but you accept the limitlessness of God as well. Something has ended, it's true, but something new has also begun. Your youth has not been ended so much as your *prolonged* youth has been interrupted—not as some bum deal that comes at the end of the party, but as your salvation from ultimate meaninglessness, your chance to put together all the things you've learned and create something good and true. Dysfunctional, obsolete patterns of thought that blocked the pathway to your higher destiny are being interrupted at last. And while you might be feeling a bit depressed that you're no longer young, you're ecstatic that you're no longer clueless.

AT JUST ABOUT THE TIME when the world seems about to literally blow up if some sane mature grown-up doesn't come in here and do something quick, a generation now reaching midlife is becoming the sane mature grown-ups.

The state of the world today is one big rite of passage for everyone, like a trip into the jungle alone to see whether or not we can survive. If we don't, then obviously we don't have what it takes. If we do, then "You're a man, my son!" Well, that's the line for half of us anyway.

Midlife today is a second puberty of sorts. The experience, including its length, is being redefined. It is a period distinctly unlike youth, yet distinctly unlike old age. It doesn't feel like a cruise to the end of our lives so much as a cruise, at last, to the *meaning* of our lives. People who were still whining "I don't know what I want to do with my life" at the age of 40 suddenly feel as if they know. You don't feel old yet, but you don't feel young anymore either.

In her book *The Longevity Factor,* Lydia Bronte writes that we've added 15 years to our lives . . . but in the middle, not at the end. We should name and claim this period as a new midlife, for indeed it *is* new. This period was not acknowledged before because it wasn't *there* in quite the way it is now. As we acknowledge the existence of this new psychological factor in the makeup of contemporary life, we build a container for otherwise dispersed, inchoate yet remarkable feelings.

We can bless and transform the midlife experience. We do this by changing our *thoughts* about it—thoughts that inform our physical cells and constitute the blueprint for our worldly experience. The work is to do two things: drop our limited thoughts and accept unlimited ones instead. Our thoughts are reflected in our experience, from the state of our bodies to the state of our world. As we reprogram our thoughts, we reprogram everything.

For women, it's become common to say that 40 is the new 30 and 50 is the new 40. I've asked myself if we just want to believe that or if it's actually true. Conveniently for me, I've decided on the latter. But it's a double-edged sword, if you think about it: On the one hand, it's an acknowledgment that we're looking so much better for longer; on the other hand, it's also an acknowledgment of how long it's taken us to finally grow up. What generations before us seemed to figure out much sooner, we've taken years to even begin to understand.

Those now maturing into midlife and beyond will not be called a "lost generation," but *will* be considered a generation that had to lose a decade or two in order to find themselves. In the end, you weren't so much wasting time as you were working through issues that previous generations hadn't had to work through. You took longer because on a psychic level, you had a lot more to do.

Don't worry if you feel like you're over the hill now. The landscape is different. We are removing the hill.

Visiting a childhood friend of mine, I saw a photograph of her from 20 years ago. The difference was dramatic, as she'd physically transformed from radiant youth to a more reserved middle age, and her face now seemed to say, "I've given up." Yet I knew the spark of her youth wasn't gone; I could still feel the fire she'd had all her life. "That's Linda," I told her, pointing at the picture. "I think you should bring her back." And I could tell from her eyes that she knew what I meant.

We know, at least intellectually, that we don't have to sink into dowdiness or resignation at midlife. Youth can give way to something else, something equally spectacular, as we are called into the next phase of our existence. We can consciously lay claim to a more glorious mid-and-later life experience than we might otherwise have had the audacity to imagine.

We can release the weight of unprocessed pain and embrace the lightheartedness of a wiser and more humble heart. We can see this not as an end-time but as a new-time. We can embrace the fact that in God there *is* no time. The new midlife is a call of the soul.

My biggest sorrow, when looking back on my youth, is how much of it I somehow missed. No matter what age we are, the key is to not miss it. As Bonnie Raitt sang like she was singing it for all of us, "Life gets mighty precious when there's less of it to waste."

My youth was full of so many miracles that I simply couldn't see at the time. But whenever I'm tempted to dwell on the ways I failed to embrace my good while young, I am reminded that the Author of my good has not run out of miracles.

That we age, if we are lucky enough to do it, is a given. *How* we age is up to us. The purpose of this book is to take a few of its issues and look them squarely in the eye, put love into some of its more fearful places, and experience miracles we might otherwise have missed.

Author's note: Throughout this book, I quote extensively from *A Course in Miracles*. The *Course* is a self-study program of spiritual psychotherapy contained in three books. It is not a religion, but rather, a psychological mind-training based on universal spiritual themes. The practical goal of the *Course* is the attainment of inner peace through the practice of forgiveness.

Chapter One

The Long and Winding Road

One day I received a couple of videotapes in the mail, containing footage of some lectures I'd given in 1988. I told my daughter I wanted her to watch them with me, to see what her mother looked and sounded like two years before she was born. I thought I was doing this for her, but soon I realized I was doing it for me. As she watched, she was mesmerized by the image of her mom not yet weighed down by years of sorrow, still light and breezy in both body and spirit. And I was sort of mesmerized myself.

A younger man I know once said to me, "I wish I could have known you when you were young," then tried to redeem himself (once he saw me wince) by saying something about how he would have liked to have known me when I had all that fire. I thought to myself, but did not say, *I still have all that fire.* What I saw looking at those videotapes was the fire he referred to, yes, but I saw something else as well. I saw a fire I needed to reclaim for myself, a fire that the world had dampened but was still mine if I wanted it—true, it was no longer flaring to the surface, but it wasn't really gone either. It was simply buried beneath layers of accumulated burdens and disappointments. The fire itself emerged from an ageless place.

Watching the tapes of my lectures, I was surprised to see my daughter so surprised. I hadn't realized that she didn't see her mother as a lighthearted woman, full of easy jokes as well as wisdom. I saw then that I'd become someone I didn't really have to be—I had descended into the dark psychic waters of a few rough years and had simply fallen for the lies I'd heard there.

What happened to me is what happens to many of us, in one way or another. Age can hit you like a truck, knocking the wind of your youth right out of you. For years you move around in reaction, seemingly defined more by what you aren't anymore than by what you are now. Yet slowly but surely, you morph into the next phase of your life—different, but not necessarily less than as opposed to more. The less or more part is up to you.

I remember buying a CD by Joni Mitchell a few years ago. The cover art is a self-portrait of her holding a glass of red wine: I sat looking at the picture for several minutes before putting on the music. And when I did, I was appalled. Nothing seemed to sound the same; I didn't hear the Joni I thought I knew. *Oh my God,* I thought, *she's lost her voice!* The high, sweet quality was gone. I, who had listened to Joni Mitchell for decades, didn't recognize the sound I heard now. For at least five minutes

I went on and on in my head about how Joni Mitchell couldn't sing anymore.

Then I started to really listen, only to realize of course that the voice that was no longer there could not compete in magnificence with the one that had taken its place. Her voice revealed a new depth now, a longing that the voice of her younger self didn't have. Somewhere between her soul and her throat, her past and her present, good pop tunes had alchemized into high art. Light and bright melodies had become deep, stark, soulful cries from the center of things. She'd moved into a place of power that is anything but *less than.* Someone already a giant seemed to have turned into a goddess.

Her path—and her changes—were meaningful to me, given my own experience. Having begun lecturing over 40 years ago, people sometimes tell me that they wish I would lecture "like in the old days." And I know what they mean. I was flip. I was funny. I was telling it like it is. But it was the *'80s,* for God's sake! It's easy enough to be light and breezy when you've never seen anything but light and never felt anything but breeze. Later, when that's no longer true—when decades more have been added to your personal repertoire of both pain and pleasure—your voice cannot *not* change. The question is, will you then lose your true voice or finally find it?

Seasons change, but all of them are spectacular. Winter is as beautiful as summer, both in nature and in us. We needn't be less compelling with age; we're simply compelling in a different way. Being where we are now, with neither shame nor apology, is what matters most. The beauty of personal authenticity can compensate for the lost beauty of our youth. At midlife, our arms aren't as voluptuous as they used to be, but we know so much more now about what we should be doing with them.

WHEN I WAS IN MY 20S I was very into "yes": Yes, I will go here; yes, I will do that. But as I got older, I got used to saying "no": No, I can't do that because my daughter is at home and I have to get back to her; no, I can't go there because I don't have the time. It seems that I stopped thinking about why I was saying it and just got into "no" as a kind of automatic response to anything outside my comfort zone. And my comfort zone began to shrink. I ultimately realized that at a certain age, too much "no" becomes poisonous. If we're not careful, we start to say "no" to life itself. And it's the "no" that ages us.

The responsibilities of a mature life often force us to focus on things that are immediately in front of us—family, work, etc.— and in that sense, "settling down" can be a good thing. But such focus doesn't have to translate into a constricted state of mind. No one can age well who lets go of their sense of wonder. You might find yourself thinking things like, *Oh, that museum. Been there, done that.* But if you make the visit anyway, you'll realize that what you saw at the museum in your younger years was only a fraction of what your eyes can see now.

If you don't exercise your body, then your muscles begin to constrict. And if you don't exercise your mind, then your attitudes begin to constrict.

Nothing constricts your life experience like the constriction of your thoughts. It limits your possibilities, and it limits your joy.

All of us have seen people who've aged with sorrow; we've seen others as well who've aged with joy. It's time to *intend* to age with joy, deciding that the joy of youth is a good kind of joy, but it's not the only kind. In fact, there is a joy in knowing that after all these years, we've finally grown up.

A wave of new possibility unfolds as the next generation reaches the years of thinning hair and less easy knee bends. What we will do at that age is not predetermined but rather remains to be seen, as every person decides, consciously or unconsciously, how to approach the chapter of midlife. We can acquiesce to the downward pull of age and chaos, or we can fearlessly forge new ground—wielding the power of what life has taught us so far, laying claim to the possibility of redemption not only for ourselves but for the entire world.

Sometimes we enter midlife feeling sort of unprepared, having partied a bit too long and matured a bit late. Yet now that there is less of it left, we're ready at last to *show up* for life. We have the knowledge, and hopefully the courage, to stand up for what we know to be true. We realize one chapter of the book of our lives has closed, but perhaps the next one doesn't have to be worse. In fact, it could be infinitely better. These years can be something to celebrate and cherish, if we have the courage to take the reins of consciousness and create something new for ourselves and for the world.

The drama of our youth doesn't diminish; it transforms. Each of us has gone through our own private dramas, taken our own individual journeys; now we meet, as though at a predestined point, to pool our resources of talent and intelligence, faith and hope. Ultimately, we are individually glorified as we find our place within a collective heartbeat. We have journeyed alone, and now we'll journey together. The real drama of this age is far from over. In a way, it's just about to begin.

EVERY GENERATION COMES bearing its own gifts as well as its own challenges. To prepare ourselves for the glorious possibilities inherent in the middle years, we need at a certain point to take stock. Entering midlife has as much to do with facing our failures, and the lessons they have taught us, as with taking credit for anything. Sometimes we feel we haven't quite yet done what we were born to do, and we are yearning to do it.

Sometimes we feel we wasted our youth, not that we lived it frivolously, but that we lived it only for ourselves. Some psychotherapeutic trends proved not to have served us well, fostering within us a dysfunctional self-reference that leaves us lonely and empty at a time when we most need the comfort of relationships. Taught to overanalyze everything we could possibly find wrong with life, we put off a more mature existence for as long as we possibly could. Now, having simmered as in a pressure cooker for decades too long, a latent lifeforce emerges with a power and sensitivity we hardly knew we had. Where we should have gotten to and what we should have realized at 20 or 30, we're getting to at 40, 50, and 60. But it's not too late. We haven't lived through what we've lived through, bled the way we've bled, and been humbled the way we've been humbled to have it just be *over* now. In fact, we owe too much to the world to get off that easily. We were all born carrying a promise—a promise to make the world better—and there's a yearning to make good on that promise that none of us can suppress forever.

There's a silent question blaring loudly in our hearts: *What will I do with the time that still stretches before me?* Perhaps we've been given a kind of reprieve, some extra time in which to get it right. Maybe because at the deepest level we were longing for one more chance to do something meaningful before we pass into eternity. Eternity might still be quite a ways away, but it's definitely time to get started.

It is the awful power of our newfound humility that gives us our one last chance at significance. Will we repudiate the glamorous meaninglessness that marked our lives until now? Will we recognize the dark and corrupting patterns of our past and rise up to change them? Will we wield the power of lessons learned? Will we align with the creative pulse of the universe, preparing the ground for a glorious future in which no one can say that we simply gave up, but everyone can say that we finally got going? Once we reach a certain point, the revolving door comes around again. We have to get it right this time or we'll die having gotten it wrong.

What we have called our "middle age" need not be a turning point toward death. It can be a turning point toward life as we have never known it, as we *could* never know it, when we were too young and arrogant to yet appreciate its limits. Aging humbles us, it's true—but it also awakens us to how precious life is, and how very fragile. It's time for us to become elders and caretakers of this precious planet, not just in name but in passionate practice. Until such time as God calls us home, we should make of *this* world the home of our dreams.

The realization that we're no longer young collides at this moment with a sense of historical urgency. Our eyes are opened to the seriousness of this time, and our deepest desire is to do something about it. As we renew our commitment to the processes of life, then the processes of life will recommit to us. We'll feel forgiven for a past that wasn't all it should have been when we commit to a future that *is* all that it can, should, and will be—now that we've finally grown up.

The prodigal son did get home late, having partied hard, but his father rejoiced to see him. And so does ours.

Wherever you've been, and whatever you've done so far, your entire life was building up to this moment. Now is the time to burst forth into your greatness—a greatness you could never have achieved without going through exactly the things you've gone through. Everything you've experienced was grist for the mill by which you have become who you are. As low as you might have descended, in God there are no limits to how high you can go now. It is *not* too late. You are *not* too old. You are right on time. And you are better than you know.

Dear God,
May every phase of my life
be blessed.
May my thoughts of fear
not block Your miracles.
May I age into a deeper love.
In this, as in all things, dear God,
may the world not blind me
to You.
Amen

Chapter Two

Do You Believe in Magic?

At a certain point, life becomes less about who you're becoming and more about who you've become. What you used to think of as the future has become the present, and you can't help but wonder if your life wouldn't be better if you'd just lived it more fully in the past. But how could you have? You were too busy thinking about the future!

Once you're past a certain age, you can hardly believe you wasted even one minute of your youth not enjoying it. And the last thing you want to do now is steal any more life from yourself by failing to be deeply in it while it's happening. You finally get it—not just theoretically, but viscerally—that this moment is all we have.

In our younger years we spent so much time trying to *be* someone. The miracle of midlife is realizing that who we are when *we're not trying to be anyone* is the someone we've been trying to be!

You don't close your eyes anymore and wonder who you might be in 20 years; if you're smart, you study the tape of your current existence to monitor how you're doing now. You see the present as an ongoing act of creation. You look more closely at your thoughts, behavior, and interaction with others. You understand that if you're coming at life from fear and separation, you have no reason to expect anything but fear and separation back. You seek to increase your strengths and decrease your weaknesses. You look at your wounds and ask God to heal them. You ask forgiveness for the things you're ashamed of. You no longer seek your satisfaction in things outside yourself, completion in other people, or peace of mind in either the past or future. You are who you *are,* not who you might one day be. Your life is what it *is,* not what it might someday be. Focusing on who you are and what your life is right now, you come to the ironic and almost amusing realization that, yes, the fun is in the journey itself.

One of my biggest regrets is missing the Christmas pageant at my daughter's preschool when she was three years old. On the one hand, someone working for me didn't bother to tell me about it; on the other, I'd obviously given off the vibe that I wouldn't care or didn't have time to go. And now I sometimes think to myself what I wouldn't give to see that pageant now. I have a memory missing, and it feels like a hole where a smile should be. It takes years—for some of us, too many years—to realize that there is nothing more precious than the look on a small child's face when they are happy to see us.

I felt ashamed when I realized that I'd become a bit like my father, who was so concerned about his career in his 40s and 50s that his emotional availability to his children was relegated to only one day of the week. During the week it was all work, work, work. On Sundays, I had him; every other day, I longed for him. Years later, when his first granddaughter came along, he'd aged to that more mellow place where being present to a child seemed at last more satisfying than being present to his work.

I used to feel jealous of the little girls whom he grandfathered with so much care and attention. I knew that if he had fathered me the way he grandfathered them, I would have become a different woman. How horrified I was years later to hear my five-year-old daughter say these pitiful words: "I miss my mommy even when she's here."

Seeing places where we have been unconscious before, we have a desire to do it all again—but *right* this time! Midlife is like this marvelous wink from God, a chance to be now who we were not before. Many people atone for not having been better parents by being much better grandparents. And that's often how their children forgive them. But some situations aren't so amenable to redoing, and some years can't so easily be made up. That's why it's so important to appreciate that the best time to try to be your best is in the present moment. You'll never have a better chance.

Dear God,
Please expand my constricted mind.
Open my clouded eyes that I might see.
Do not allow me to escape my good.
Help me not to miss my life.
Prepare my heart for better things.
Amen

One day I looked at myself in the mirror and indulged in full-scale self-pity.

Oh, I remember when I was young, I thought. My skin was tighter, my breasts were higher, my rear was firmer, my entire body was voluptuous. I had so much more energy, and I practically glowed. I wish I had realized what I had when I had it . . . and now I'll never have it again.

Then another voice in my head intervened.

"Oh, Marianne . . . ," it said, *"shut up! Let me give you a rundown of what it was like when you were younger. Your nerves were shot, your heart was restless, your mind was disordered, your appetites were addictive, your love affairs were tragic, your talents were squandered, your opportunities were wasted, and you were never at peace.*

"What you did then, in fact, was exactly what you're doing now: You kept thinking that if only things were different, you'd be happy. Then it was whatever man or job or resources were there to save you; now it's if only you were still young. Reality check: In those days, you looked good, but you didn't know it. You had everything, but you didn't appreciate it. You had the world at your feet, but you didn't realize it.

"You know what it was like, Marianne? It was just like now!"

Thus began my recovery from "youth-itis." I still slipped back into it every once in a while, but as time went on, I would snap out of it faster and faster. I realize it's nothing more than a mental habit to idealize another time, another condition, another reality—as simply a way to avoid the reality of my life right now.

And in avoiding the reality of our present circumstances, we blind ourselves to the miracles that are all around us. One of my biggest character weaknesses, I've discovered, is that I tend to show up too late for things. Whether it was a city, or a relationship, or a professional opportunity, I would take too much time before I really *got* there. My mind would be on the past, or the future, or whatever else seemed more important at the time than simply being fully present for what was available now. And by the time I finally did show up, not everybody was still all that interested. We miss out on so many things not because they aren't happening, but simply because *we* weren't happening. We go around bemoaning lack of opportunity, when the deeper work is how to realize how many opportunities came and went because we didn't take advantage of them. These are the kinds of things that make midlife a new beginning: a chance to get it right in areas where, when we were younger, we got it wrong.

Midlife is the time to stare down this self-defeating habit and cultivate a truer perspective: Wherever we are is the perfect place, and whatever time it is now is the perfect time. Show up for how you look *now*! Show up for what you can do *now*! Show up for the people who are in front of you *now*! Indulging the thought that *if only we were younger, things would be better* is 1) a lie, and 2) a surefire way to age with pain.

MY FATHER ONCE TOLD ME, "When you're old, you don't feel old." I can appreciate what he meant when he said that, as I ponder the fact that the essential being I am inside myself is the same in my 50s as when I was only 15. So who am I really? Am I the woman who has changed with age, or am I the changeless self within? Am I a woman who is encased in time or the being who dwells apart from it?

Sometimes when referring to things that happened long ago, we say things like "I remember it like it was yesterday." And that's because in a way it was. If time, as Einstein declared, is merely an illusion of consciousness, then linear time itself is a metaphysical fiction; everything that has happened, is happening, or will happen, is happening *now.* There, in that realm of the eternal now, is the true "I am."

The eternal self dwells in eternity, and eternity intersects linear time at only one point: the present. Who you are in this moment, therefore, is who you truly are. And who you are is love itself. From that essential point of perfect being, created anew by God every instant, miracles flow naturally. Love interrupts the past and opens the future to new probabilities. No matter who you are, no matter how old you are, in the present, all things are possible.

The physical self ages, of course, but the spiritual self does not. As we identify more with the spiritual dimension of our lives, then our experience begins to shift from the changeable to the changeless . . . from limitation to limitlessness . . . from fear to love. As our journey through linear time gets shorter, our consciousness can in fact expand. And as it does, time itself is affected. The deeper we go into the love at the heart of things, the more we actualize our earthly potential. The understanding of that which does *not* change is the key to our power within a world that does. In aligning ourselves with the eternal Self, we age not in a straight line leading from voluptuous youth to decrepit age, but rather like the flowering lotus opening more and more to the light of the sun. And age becomes a miracle.

Physically, we get older and then we die. Yet spiritually, whether we go backward or forward is a matter not of the body but of consciousness. When we think about age differently, then our experience of age changes. We can be physically older but emotionally and psychologically younger. In the words of Emily Dickinson, "We turn not older with years but newer every day."

Some of us were in a state of decay in our 20s and are in a state of rebirth in our 60s or 70s. King Solomon, who supposedly was the wisest of all men, described his youth as his winter and his advanced years as his summer. We can be older than we used to be yet feel much younger than we are.

As we become more spiritually intelligent, more aware of the forces that underlie and cause all earthly reality, then issues of age begin to transform. This isn't just metaphysical jargon; it's a description of how consciousness operates. Spiritual growth increases our sense of what's possible. And as we *sense* new possibility, we can *step into* that possibility. With every word, every thought, every action, we choose what we wish to call forth in life. Old thoughts create old scenarios, and we can choose to let them go.

According to *A Course in Miracles,* we achieve so little because our minds are undisciplined. We're too easily lured into self-deprecating thoughts, limited beliefs, and negative self-perception. No one *forces* you to think, *My best years are behind me,* or *No one will want me anymore,* or *I missed my chance.* But whatever it is you choose to think, your subconscious mind takes it very seriously and your experience will reflect your thinking.

Our very cells respond to the thoughts we think—with every word, silent or spoken, we participate in the body's functioning. We participate in the functioning of the universe itself. If our consciousness grows lighter, then so does everything within and around us.

This means, of course, that with every thought, you can start to re-create your life.

AT MIDLIFE, YOU SUDDENLY SEE AN ENDGAME where you used to see an endless stretch. You know now on a visceral level that this lifetime will not go on forever. There's no more time for five-year detours. No more time for getting it wrong. No more time for relationships that don't serve, or for staying in situations that aren't authentically you. No more time for playing small, false pride, or whatever other roadblock emerged from the dark waters of your psyche to obstruct the joy that's meant to be yours. You want to become a precision instrument now—focusing on exactly what you want to do and being exactly who you need to be.

According to ancient Asian philosophy, time is not a line but a spiral. Every life lesson that has ever been presented to us (which means everything we have ever been through) will come back again, in some form, until we learn it. And the stakes each time will be higher. Whatever we've learned will bear greater fruit. Whatever we've failed to learn will bear harsher consequences.

Whatever *didn't* work in your life before this point was a reflection of the fact that you hadn't yet integrated the different parts of yourself. Where you didn't yet accept yourself, you attracted a lack of acceptance in others. Where you hadn't yet dealt with your shadows, you manifested shadowy situations. Broken parts of you encountered broken parts of others. So now you know! That was then and this is now.

Midlife is our second chance. If you want to spend the years you have left simply reenacting the dramas of your past, you can. The same script will indeed be coming around again for your review. It always does. But if you choose, you can take the script and give it an awesome rewrite, totally get on top of your material, and take a bow at the end that blows everyone away.

Your play might be set in another town this time and the characters might be different. But it is essentially the same play. Whether you were ready for your starring role last time is another story. Whether you behaved in a way that welcomed your opportunities and maximized their benefits is another story. But the fact that you ever attracted opportunities in the first place means that they belonged to you. They are encoded in your script. Now—through the power of your atonement, humility, and a sincere desire to get it right in areas where you might have gotten it wrong before—you will attract the same opportunities again, in another form. An all-merciful God will send them around once more, with even bigger plans for how they can bless you and others now.

Do the rewrite carefully. Your character should not say "I'm too old now," but rather "I'm just getting started." "I'm too weak for this" can be "I am strong now." "I blame them for what they did to me" can be "I choose to forgive." "What can I get from this situation?" can be "What can I contribute?" "I have to pretend to be someone other than I am" can be "Who I am is already good enough." "What do I think I should do?" can be "Dear God, what would You have me do?" With every new thought, you can work a miracle—changing your script and changing your life.

Dear God,
I wish to change my life,
so please, dear God,
change me.
Remove from my mind all judgment
and from my heart all fear.
Release the chains that bind me
and free me to my truer Self.
Increase my faith in the spirit
You have placed in me.
Amen

I remember an experience at a restaurant my family frequented when I was a child. Its backyard garden was decorated in a magical way at night, full of bubbles and multicolored lights. I felt sure there were otherworldly beings cavorting by the fountain, and while others around me ate dinner and talked, I sat mesmerized by the view. An entire drama unfolded outside the window, a fairyland scenario acted out on a stage of light that only I could see.

Decades later, I can still see it.

As children we loved such things, but then we grew up and were told they're just fantasies to be left behind. We were indoctrinated into a disenchanted world, and we've sacrificed a lot in order to live there. The world isn't better off for having forfeited its tenderness. The meanness and cynicism of our age, the reflexive sarcasm that passes for intelligent reflection, the suspicion and judgment of everyone and everything—such are the toxic by-products of a disenchanted worldview.

In our hearts we want off that wheel of suffering. We don't want to accept that *what is* is *what has to be.* We want to pierce the veil of illusion that separates us from a world of infinite possibility. We want another kind of life—for ourselves and for the world—and the hunger to find it becomes more intense as we grow older.

At midlife we're at a fork in the road: We either accept the modern materialist's view of the world, in which case we just keep on truckin' until we finally die; or we consider that our visit to a disenchanted world was simply an error—the archetypal exile from the Garden of Eden. Now we can return to at least some semblance of the Garden if we choose. Perhaps the enchantment of our childhood perspective was not so much fantasy as a not-truly-lost reality that can still be reclaimed. Perhaps there is a door to miraculous realms that is simply waiting for us to open it.

We can consider that there might be another way. And when we do, we recognize our responsibility to claim it—for ourselves and for the world.

Today is much like ancient times, when people carrying the "old" wisdom were overrun by the encroachments of the early church. Today it is not an institution that holds us down. The oppressor is simply a mistaken, patriarchal worldview, a monster with many heads that posits a world where the forces of the soul (and women) are peripheral. No matter what form this oppressor takes, or where it comes from, the only point that matters is that you can believe whatever you want to believe. And what you believe will be true for you.

We've been brainwashed and misled by the prejudices of modernity. A rationalistic, mechanistic worldview eradicated several colors on the color wheel and then pronounced itself better eyesight. Increasing our capacity in some areas of the brain, it diminished our capacity in others. While we have mapped the outer territories of the world—from outer space to the tiny atom—we're only crudely aware of the parallel universe of the inner self. And how can you navigate a land you refuse to see?

If you want to believe that what your physical eyes can see is all that's there, then fine, go ahead. Stay in that small fraction of perceptual reality if you choose. But at some point—even if that point is at the point of death—we all know better. I've seen cynics become mystics on their deathbeds. We are here as if in a material dream, from which the spiritual nature of our larger reality is calling us to awaken. The magician, the alchemist, the miracle worker, is simply someone who has woken up to the material delusions of the world and decided to live another way. In a world gone mad, we can choose to be sane.

In order to move ourselves—and our civilization—into the next phase of our evolutionary journey, it's time to reenchant ourselves. The wizard Merlin was an old man with a long white beard. He wasn't born a full-fledged wizard so much as he *became* a full-fledged wizard. And his becoming, like yours and mine, would have taken years. Most of us have ventured away from the knowing in our hearts, and what we encountered on our detour had deep significance. The mystical kingdom of sorcerers and castles, brave knights and dragons, turns out to be a more mature rendition of our soul's journey than anything the so-called realists ever taught us.

Children's fairy tales aren't fantasy so much as an archetypal road map. It's our modern worldview that represents fantasy—the fantasy that the world revealed to us by our physical senses is all that is—and finally seeing that, applying its truths, is the key to midlife awakening.

IN *BEAUTY AND THE BEAST*, a beautiful prince turns into a horrible beast—until unconditional love turns him back into who he really is. Gee, that sounds like almost everyone I know.

Years ago, after my first book was published, my lawyer recounted to me a conversation he'd had with my publisher. The publisher had made a comment about my being a "spiritual teacher," to which my lawyer replied, "She's not! She writes books about spirituality, but she's not a spiritual teacher." I remember wanting to say, "Actually, John, I think I *am* a spiritual teacher," but I didn't, out of fear that it would appear immodest. Who was I to call myself that? Yet as it says in *A Course in Miracles,* we create what we defend against; in an effort to dissuade people from thinking I thought of myself as any big deal, I acted in a way that ensured they would.

Oh, you think I'm so spiritual? Watch this! I can be stupid, too! Thinking it was humble to do so, I dissociated who I was when I wasn't working from the more enlightened persona that came naturally to me when I was. The ego defends the "separate self," leading to thoughts that lead to behavior that often reflect our "opposite." That is what many of us are doing in this life: living the opposite of our truth, just as the beast was the opposite of the beautiful prince in the fairy tale.

We prance around on a stage of illusion, acting out whatever pathetic bit part the fear-based ego allows us in this tragic play, repeating our lines without realizing this isn't the script with which we came into this life. Our script, in fact, got switched at birth—we're playing a part that is not our part and repeating lines that are not our lines.

The ego not only defends against our expressing our true selves, but also against our consciously seeing that this is what we're doing. Our opposite becomes the personality that we, and everyone else, thinks we actually are. Then, since the ego is guiding how we're presenting ourselves, the world comes to agree that of course that *is* who we actually are. We're no longer princes, but beasts. And thus we are double bound: first by appearing as not who we really are, and then by the dark contagion of a world that is judging us for it.

It's a radical epiphany to finally realize that exactly who we are is quite enough. To accept that God has given each of us a magnificent role to play on Earth merely because we're human; that we were born with a perfect script etched on our hearts; that it's not to our personal credit, but to His greater glory, that each of us is brilliant—such are the truths that free us from the ego's lies. Mystical understanding is a ray of light, God's kiss that transforms us back into who we truly are. Each of us can put down the burden of our false self and allow our truth to reemerge.

The world in which we live today—reflecting in so many ways the opposite of our sweetness and love—reminds us how desperately important it is to break the spell that's been cast on the human race and retrieve our shining Self. Our inner sweetness—whether we call it "the Christ," "the soul," or whatever word describes the spiritual essence so not at home in our worldly zones of combat—is the only place where we will ever, ever, be safe. The outer kingdom is not our real home. The inner kingdom is our everything. And until we retrieve it, our outer kingdom will be a land of suffering for everyone.

My dreamlike and mystical nature as a child could rarely find acceptance within my family system or support at school, a conundrum to which I responded—as most people do to the stress of finding ourselves psychologically housed where we are not at home—by psychically splitting off from myself. I separated from my authentic spirit, thinking I needed to be someone else. My spirit wandered high above me, like in novels where an elderly family member is relegated to the attic so as not to be an embarrassment to the rest of the family. What I didn't realize, of course, was that she who was exiled was the beauty within, and without her I was bereft without knowing why.

The split I experienced was not unusual. It's the destiny of everyone born into this world to lose ourself, then try to find ourself again. The split commonly begins in our teenage years and becomes acute in our 20s. From that point forward a painful confusion can continue to plague us. By midlife, a desperate sense of loss—often having been temporarily assuaged by various forms of dysfunctional attachment to people, events, or substances—leads, if we're fortunate, to the spiritual realization that "By God, what I was looking for was me all along."

I remember when I was a little girl, one of my friends lived in a house where there was a mural painted on the wallpaper in the powder room. It showed two little angels lying on clouds holding hand mirrors. And that powder room at Beth Klein's house became like a chapel to me. I would come up with any excuse to enter that bathroom and just stare up at the mural. I felt like it was speaking to me of something; now, of course, I realize it was a realm I had been in and longed to reclaim. I wondered if others could see what I could see on that wall of my Sistine Chapel on Tartan Lane.

How young we were, so many of us, when we were spiritually cast away from ourselves. Having felt cast out, we collectively manifested a world from which, if we don't change things quickly, we *will* be cast out. The only way we can fundamentally heal a situation in which the human race teeters on the brink of all manner of catastrophe is to repair the original separation between who we truly are and the imposters we're tempted to become become.

At midlife, we get that. *Beauty and the Beast* is the story of the soul. The Beast is the part of ourselves that split off from who we truly are; Beauty is the part of ourselves that comes to our own rescue.

In the words of poet T. S. Eliot:

> We shall not cease from exploration
> And the end of all our exploring
> Will be to arrive where we started
> And know the place for the first time.

Every life is a microcosm of the greater global drama. As each of us returns to the truth in our hearts, we will be released to our highest creativity and intelligence. This will open up avenues of repair the mortal mind can't even imagine, leading us to co-create with God a transformed experience of life on earth. Realigned within ourselves, we will realign the world. And heaven and earth shall be as one.

IN 2007, HAVING BEEN READING *A Course in Miracles* for three decades and lecturing on it literally thousands of times, I came out of meditation one day and thought, *I've become an advanced student of the Course!* Not an advanced *practitioner,* mind you, but an advanced student. And that took 30 years.

What is it about spiritual knowledge that takes so long to digest? The trendy nature of much contemporary seeking would lead you to think that you spend a year or two at the ashram and *voilà!*—you're at the mountaintop. But my experience argues otherwise. It takes a decade to understand the basic nature of spiritual principles, another decade while the ego tries to eat you alive, another decade while you try to wrestle it to the ground, and finally you begin to walk more or less in the light. Anyone who thinks a spiritual path is easy probably hasn't been walking one.

What does all this mean: to embrace the light, walk in the light, and so on? What is all this light, light, light talk? In *A Course in Miracles,* light is defined as "understanding." What a beautiful thought, that to see the light is to understand.

By midlife, we're usually aware enough to understand which of our issues most need attention. We've learned where we're strong, but also where we're weak. We know what parts of ourselves to be proud of and what parts need to change. We know what our *issues* are this lifetime. It might not be a time when we're learning *new* things about ourselves, so much as a time to understand more deeply what we already know. And new levels of self-awareness bring new opportunities for breakthrough.

This is not the time to stop working on ourselves; it's the time when we've finally accumulated enough clues to help crack the case and solve the mystery of why and how we've kept ourselves bound for so long. It's not the time to give up and say, "This is just how I am. It's too late to change." Quite the opposite—it's time to take a stand, once and for all, for your own potential. Don't worry that it took you so long to get to this point. It takes everyone this long. We know nothing until we know all the ways that we're not who we should be. Only then do we have a chance at becoming the people we've wanted to be, and God intended us to be, from the day we were born.

For that reason alone, these are sacred years.

You can't really build a life till you've pulled together all the things you've finally come to understand about yourself. And life would be cruel if at just about the time you've finally started to figure it out, it reached some sort of predetermined disintegration. Just as adolescents must separate from their parents, you need to separate from the person you were before this point, to whatever extent that person was not the real you.

Finding out who we actually aren't, we begin to understand at last who we actually are.

In my book ILLUMINATA, I wrote a midlife rite of passage to mark the end of one phase of life and the beginning of another. Such rituals are important markers in a person's journey, reminding not only us but those around us to honor what has been before and to embrace what now can be.

Dear God,
Please soften my heart
where it has hardened.
Please help me reach
for higher thoughts.
Please pave the way
for a better life
for me and all the world.
Amen

THOSE OF US WHO HAVE EXPERIENCED THE MOST—its good as well as its bad—have greater knowledge of the beasts of chaos and unruliness that threaten the earth today. We've learned the hard way that the darkness of the world is a reflection of the darkness inside us. We'll learn to tame the beast of the world by taming it within ourselves.

When we're young, we're powerful in a physical sense. The strength of youth is not earned so much as given to you as a gift from nature. It serves a role that belongs specifically to the young: to procreate and build external structures that support material life.

Ralph Waldo Emerson said, "As we grow old, the beauty steals inward." And so does ours. But we're responsible for make it visible. We can still be beautiful, but in a different kind of way. And the beauty of age isn't simply given to us, as it was in our youth; it has to be earned. And it is often earned as much through suffering as through joy. Our failures as well as our successes, if processed and alchemized into the stuff of true character, can ultimately strengthen rather than weaken us. Our physical muscles cannot carry the weight of the world's emotional pain—only spiritual musculature, often built through accumulated repetitions of heartache, can do that. This isn't a deficiency in nature's plan, but an economy in nature's plan. We weren't being beaten down; we were being honed.

And if we're willing to accept it, age endows us with a spiritual elixir. Having seen the darkness in ourselves and others, we've become more humble before the light. Having been brought out of darkness, we've developed a devotion to He Who delivered us. Having made serious mistakes, we know how much forgiveness matters. Having suffered, we feel more compassion for the suffering of others. They're not just abstractions to us anymore; they are principles that have infused our flesh. *And they are the very things that make us more beautiful.* They were not our defeats but our victories. We are strong now in ways we could not have been before. And our strength is needed. We are entering a time when our internal strengths, more than our external ones, will be humanity's most important sources of renewal and repair. Layers of false power have given way to something far more real.

Whatever powers we might lose with age are small compared to the powers we stand to gain. There's a profound satisfaction in finally giving up something meaningless, for no other reason than that we did it to the max and now we're ready to move on. Midlife is about surrendering things that no longer matter, not because our lives are in decline but because they're on an *incline*. Traveling upward, we simply let go of some baggage. Maybe there's more natural wisdom in what's happening to us now than we think. Of all those things we can't remember, is it possible that any of them are completely unimportant? Could it be that nature is *demanding* rather than just requesting that we simplify? The only way we can peacefully age is if we have respect for the demands of the experience.

It's almost embarrassing to admit, but sometimes it's a relief to get to finally slow down. You realize "slower" is not necessarily "worse than." The speed of our former years was not as constructive as it appeared to be. Moving too fast, we often missed a lot. Many of us made big mistakes we might not have made if we hadn't been moving through life so quickly.

I remember when I was young hearing Otis Redding sing, "Sitting here resting my bones . . . ," and thinking, *Who needs to rest their bones?* Now of course I know. And when I first had the thought one day that I was just sitting there resting my bones, I panicked. I thought it was all over if my *bones* were tired! But then I realized something else, like a guilty secret: I was *enjoying* just sitting there. I wasn't attending a Buddhist retreat *trying* to enjoy just sitting; I really *was* enjoying it! I was enjoying the kinetic experience of a rocking chair in a way I had never thought possible. ("Oh, these things are actually *helpful!* Who knew?") I didn't feel the need to get up, to go somewhere else, or to do anything at all. With less adrenaline came less distraction. I felt no need to justify my existence by achieving or performing a thing. And that's when I realized, *This is very different, but it isn't bad.*

Sometimes what we appear to have lost is simply something it was time to leave behind. Perhaps our system just lets something go, our having moved through the experience and now needing it no more. A friend of mine was sitting once with two of his best friends, a couple he'd partied long and hard with during the 1960s. At about 10 in the evening, the couple's 20-something daughter came home, saw them on the couch, and admonished them, "You guys are so boring! You never go out!" To which all three responded in unison, "We were out, and now we're in."

The mind is its own kind of dance floor. What a mature generation could do from our rocking chairs could literally rock the world. If in fact the highest, most creative work is the work of consciousness, then in slowing down we're not doing less; we're doing *more*. Having slowed down physically, we're in a better space to rev up psychically. We are becoming contemplative. We are shifting from the outer to the inner not in order to begin our demise, but to reseed and regreen the consciousness of the planet. And that's what is happening now: We're going slower in order to go deeper, in order to go faster in the direction of urgently needed change.

Dear God,
When I rest
may I rest in You.
Transform my weariness
into readiness for something new.
I open my heart
and pray for Your guidance.
At last, I am ready
to change.
Amen

TO THE EGO, SIMPLIFICATION MEANS HAVING LESS; to the spirit, simplification means having more. Wherever there is an overabundance of material substance, our availability to Spirit is limited. Whether it's decluttering your house or dropping toxic relationships, anything you do to prune away dysfunctional material involvement leaves the soul more free to fly up to its natural state. As we approach the mountaintop of spiritual progress, we begin the process of letting go.

Age involves a lot of letting go—of some of our physical prowess, perhaps, or certain worldly opportunities, or even our children to live their own lives. Yet such letting go isn't meant to constitute a depressing sacrifice of happiness. Anytime we're called to let go of something, there's a hidden treasure to be found in the experience. Rarely does a birthing of anything new in ourselves not involve a dying of the old.

You're carefree before becoming a parent, in a way you will never be again. But you're *satisfied,* having become one, in a way you never could have been before. That's just one example of the kinds of transitions that often mark midlife. For all kinds of reasons, we're no longer carefree. But the miracle is that we're something else instead. We are grown-ups in the deepest sense, and that is new psychological and spiritual ground.

You can't remember the day when you crossed over the border from who you were to who you are, but you definitely did. The lightness of your youth is gone, perhaps, but so is your youthful suffering. Mature angst is different than youthful angst; it seems less tortured. You know too much now to either laugh *or* cry the way you used to. You see things from a different perspective, and with that new perspective has come a new sense of self. On some essential level, you are birthing a new you.

There's little in life more satisfying than the feeling that at last you've taken ownership of yourself. You don't have to be afraid anymore that some part of you—some fractal not yet integrated into your personality—is going to trip you up. You feel at last like you *inhabit* yourself. You finally went into all the rooms, turned the lights on, and settled in.

How interesting it is that the spirit should begin to open up as the body begins to slow down. It's very humbling to watch the body age. The arc of human history is coded into our cells: our bones, muscles, organs, and reproductive systems are all moving into a different mode at midlife, in an unmistakable drive toward hopefully distant but eventual death. Yet there is much we can do to enliven the body—including enlivening the mind.

We can in many ways transform the forces of death into renewed and sanctified life.

We can treat our bodies not as things that are slowly failing us, but as our partners in rebirth. If we identify only with the material world, then age creeps into us like an unwanted guest who's come to stay. But if we identify also with our spiritual existence, then our attitude toward the body becomes one of deep appreciation and gratitude. It's the house our spirit lives in, after all. When we walk, bike, do yoga, lift weights, eat correctly, take herbs and vitamins, or do whatever we can in order to treat the body well, we're not just delaying death; we're affirming life and consciously creating its next chapter. With every stretch of the body, we help stretch the mind. With every stretch of the mind, we help stretch the body. And one stretch at a time, we're renewing them both.

According to spiritual literature, the body will be with us for as long as it serves the function of the soul for us to remain here. When I was a younger woman, I took my body so for granted. In midlife, I began to feel more grateful for it, and to God for giving it to me.

There's something about having less of something—less energy, less time, less whatever—that creates a poignant shift in our sense of its value. The body *is* a miracle, after all. It seems to me that with age should come a greater willingness to treat it lovingly and with care. Your body deserves some kindness after all it's been through. And probably you do too.

Dear God,
Resanctify my body
that it might be healed and whole.
Pour forth Your Spirit
into my flesh.
May every cell receive new life,
That I might serve You more.
Amen

Chapter Three

The Nick of Time

You arrive at midlife having collected some important clues about yourself. The mission now is to discover what they mean.

Many, if not most, of our personal issues begin in childhood, most specifically within our family of origin. Young adulthood is often the time of a big escape, as we seek to evade our issues by evading our families. Ultimately, we come to realize that only by facing those issues head-on can we escape their consequences throughout our lives.

My own family has been a complicated puzzle with some oddly shaped psychological pieces. For years, my primary response to whatever discomfort I experienced there was to go live elsewhere and not return except for a quick hello every few months. I don't think I could have done otherwise, given who I was when I was younger. But having reached another stage in my life, I then realized that everything I went out into the world to find, everything I thought my family didn't have or couldn't show me, was pretty much right there in front of me all the time.

Our family is usually a microcosm of the world we'll encounter, whether we travel great distances or barely stray from home. The lessons to be learned in life have to do with the fragility of the human heart and the nobility of the human spirit; the suffering involved in simply being human and the struggles to survive the experience; the joy and laughter when our children are well; and the tears and sadness when love and lives are over. I never had to leave home to learn all this. But if you'd told me that when I was young, I wouldn't have believed you.

Whether your childhood was good or not so good, it lives in your cells. It laid down tracks of thought, and thus behavior, that have run your life for decades. If you were appreciated, you've attracted people who appreciate you. If you were unappreciated, you've attracted people who don't appreciate you. You've subconsciously been drawn to individuals and situations that mirror pretty perfectly the drama of your childhood.

In the words of novelist William Faulkner, "The past is not dead. In fact, it's not even past." Until we address the deeper drama of our past, we are bound to reenact it. The more we ignore our childhood wounds, the more they fester and grow. Until we heal the child we used to be, the adult we want to be doesn't stand a chance.

We can help release the drama of our childhood by redefining whose child we are. We are products of our family of origin, to be sure. But who is that, exactly—our mortal parentage, or our immortal one? It's an important issue because we inherit the riches of whomever we think sourced us. We might have inherited limitation and fear from our mortal parents, but we inherited miracles and love from God. Our worldly parents might have been wonderful people or they might have been scoundrels, but the larger point is that they're not who created us. Superman was only *raised* by those nice people in Kansas. His real Father was from somewhere else . . . and so is ours.

As long as we think our biological parents fundamentally sourced us, we'll feel the need to distance ourselves from them because on some level, we know it's not true. When we see that in fact they're simply fellow souls who gave us a tremendous gift by bringing us into this world, then (hopefully) did their best to take care of us and raise us right, we realize the significance of the debt we owe them. Understanding that God is our true Father/Mother, and all humanity our brothers and sisters, counterintuitively delivers us to a more, not less, respectful attitude toward our biological family. Knowing more deeply who they are in our lives—and who they aren't—frees us to love them more.

Many people today never experienced an appropriate break from their parents, remaining in the psychic grip of childhood long past the time when adulthood arrived. In the absence of a healthy rite of passage, perhaps you subconsciously created for yourself whatever drama, however painful, would force you into a more mature mode of living.

Today, we're all being forced to grow up. Both individually and collectively, we're being challenged by world events to match our talents with compassion, our intelligence with humility, and our intellect with wisdom. The grace period of youth is over for all of us. We are children no longer. We're at the front of the line.

AN IDEA YOU MIGHT FIND HELPFUL as you enter midlife, or find yourself moving through it and want to make it a more meaningful experience, is to ritualize it with a Rite of Passage.

You gather some friends or family—only those who appreciate the significance of the event, by the way, and will bring the fullness of themselves to the experience. You owe it to yourself to not make your heart available to trivialization of any kind as you prepare for this.

In my book *Illuminata*, I wrote a ceremony that you might find of interest. Or you can write your own. Like the baptism of a child, a Bar or Bat Mitzvah, a wedding, or even a funeral, sacred rites are psychological portals that prepare not only an individual but also the community around them for the healthiest journey into what comes next.

And much *will* come next. Midlife is a fundamental change, and one that presages others. The more we accept that changes are inevitable, we open to receive them rather than trying to distance ourselves from the feelings they bring up for us. Whether we age is rarely our decision. Whether we age *happily* is very much so. Even in the happiest life we have some unhapppy days. And once we reach midlife, there are layers of loss that become more commonplace.

A frequent experience of loss at midlife is the declining health, or death, of our parents. Those who brought us into the world are usually the ones to leave it first. They welcomed us when we got here; now we'll wish them farewell as they move on to the next phase of their souls' journey.

When I was younger, I couldn't bear the thought of my father dying. And that was a persistent terror throughout my earlier years. How would I continue to exist if he were not here? Yet the anticipation of someone's death is often far worse than the feelings we experience once it's happened; I found that Daddy's having died was far less excruciating than the *fear* that he would. With my father's passing, and then with my sister's, I never felt that my immediate family dwindled from five members to three. Rather, it's as if there's a photograph of five people in my head, and two of them are photographic negatives. But the picture is the same. They're still my family.

My father was a profoundly charismatic person. Yet with that came shadows, as is often the case. With him taking such a starring role in the family drama, who else had a chance to play as large a part as we might have otherwise? I've noticed something similar with my daughter, how she herself has handled a situation where the parent is not exactly a shrinking violet. I've always felt she made a preverbal decision: She could either let Mom be the star here and simply accept the role of background player; or she could come out blazing in the first act, making it very clear to everyone that this would be an ensemble drama, thank you. Lord knows she chose the latter. And I say, *Good for her.*

I hope she will have plenty of experience starring in her own life long before I leave. So far she certainly is, and I'm thrilled to applaud her. Yet in my case, and in the case of many people, we don't really have an experience of starring in our own lives until at least one parent has left the stage.

It's not until you're in the generation that will be leaving next that you feel the full weight and power of being the star in your own life. So it is that while we feel the sadness of our parents' aging and grieve for them when they pass away, we also know—as my father used to tell me—that death is part of a greater mystery. When I think of him now, I smile at the thought that he's no longer an old man. Someone told me once that when you die, the spirit goes back to being 35. Of course it's preposterous to think that anyone really knows these things. It's sort of like the question "If someone I love reincarnates, does that mean they won't be there to meet me on the other side when I arrive?" Who the hell knows.

But I know this: After he died, I *felt* my father. I could have sworn he said to me, very slowly, "Oh, *that's* who you are!" Clearly, he had not fully seen me when he was here. But once he was gone, I felt that he could. And I can feel he does. As much as he did for me as a father, there were limits to what he could do because there were limits to what he could see. But his dying didn't end our relationship; we've simply entered the next phase of it. And what he has given me since, in the purity of spirit, more than makes up for what he withheld from me when he was living. My father didn't simply get old and then die. In the end, after his death, he became to me even more of who he is.

And so did I.

Dear God,
Please heal my relationship with my parents.
Whether they're on Earth
or have passed beyond the veil of death,
may only love remain between us.
May I not be broken by their weaknesses,
but may I be strengthened by their strengths.
May they be at peace,
and so may I.
Help me to forgive them,
That I might be healed.
Amen

In youth, we encounter our psychic dragons; by midlife, it's time to slay them. It's the time for a major commitment to heal whatever childhood wounds remain. There can be no spiritual victory without this.

It's not as hard to heal from these patterns as we sometimes think, once we're honest with ourselves about (l) what they are, and (2) who's 100 percent responsible for them. A wound that might have been inflicted on you years ago by someone else has turned into a character defect that is all yours now. No matter who might have caused your problem when you were a child, you're responsible for it as an adult. To the extent that we project responsibility for a dysfunction outside ourselves, we cannot change it. Wherever our wound came from, however many years ago, its healing lies not in the past but in the present. Your subconscious will continue to trigger the wound for as long as it takes—a 50-year-old experiencing a 5-year-old's pain—until you make a stand for your own healing.

And that takes courage, because it means we have to look at our stuff. Really, really, really look at it. If at midlife we do not do that, dysfunctional psychological patterns begin to harden; self-sabotaging emotional habits will trip us up even more and more often. Counterintuitively, the longer they remain with us, the less we can see them. A blind spot is called a blind spot for exactly that reason; we are blind to it. Midlife is the time to fess up to ourselves, to take the courageous look in the mirror that our ego would rather we not do. To look at problems in our lives and recognize that we ourselves were the common element. We have lived enough to see the ways we have blown it when we have blown it, and this is the time to decide to change.

There is no more powerful way to change a bad habit than to ask God to take it away. The Spirit of God works through our subconscious mind, literally impressing itself on the wiring of our brain. That's the ultimate meaning of the line that "In the beginning was the Word."

Every word forms a thought, and every thought creates form on some level. The altar to God is in your mind; placing a situation on the altar means asking that your thoughts about it be altered. Thought is the level of Cause, as your world is the level of Effect. Asking God to heal something means you are asking for transformation on the causal level, that the effects in your life might change.

When you ask God to help you change something in your life, you're asking that your subconscious mind bring into your awareness every thought that will help you do that.

That's the spiritual reality behind the "consciousness work" so popular today. When Divine Intelligence and human intelligence align as one, we reprogram not only our own awareness but also the state of the world. As we mature, our accumulated experiences have proven what merely abstract theory could not. *Oh I get it now, when I blew that relationship I wasn't in my right mind. My fear overcame my love. If I had prayed before that conversation, I would not have said such a ridiculous thing.* We begin to realize that spirituality has very practical application. We're ready at last to apply what in our younger years we might have known, but we didn't *really* yet know. And that becomes our gift to the world: having been to hell and back, we can help save others the bother.

We've learned it takes more than psychological insight to heal our childhood wounds. We need to do more than analyze the past; we need to forgive it. And we must surrender the idea that the world around us should accommodate our pain. Should we not do those things, we age but we do not mature. There is something subtly pathetic about a woman in midlife who hasn't cleared the issues that everyone deals with in our 20s. The beauty of midlife and beyond is not that we haven't suffered, but that we have transformed our suffering in a way that makes us stronger. That is our beauty stolen inward.

Men and women live in a different emotional universe than little boys and girls. It's sad when a child doesn't get the chance to experience childhood. But it's pathetic when an adult never gets around to being an adult. Children are victims, but adults have the tools to embrace a victory. An adult still acting from a childish place might say, "I'm needy because my parents abandoned me; the right partner will understand that!" The true adult knows better, and is hardly looking for someone to cater to their wounds. The adult knows their perfect partner is someone who has compassion for our wounds but doesn't acquiesce to needy behavior. He or she says firmly and sincerely, "I'm genuinely sorry you went through that. Now get over it."

Why? Because we have a purpose in midlife. We emerge from the cocoon of chronic self-reference and show up to help heal the world. We have tools with which to do that that we might not have had before. Maturity is a mantle that makes us more, not less, powerful. It's the crowning achievement of having gone through what we've gone through and made it through to the other side.

Yet what do we do with those childhood wounds? Is there a spiritual solution to the ways in which we sabotage our lives, keeping us stuck in immaturity and angst at a time when our souls are prepared to move on to higher ground? When the spirit is ready to break free of the chains of past pain, yet we psychologically and emotionally remain in its grip, our most powerful tool is to ask God for help. "Dear God, I act so (blank) that it's destroying my relationships. Please heal me and show me a better way to be." Prayer is the medium of miracles. It will activate our power to change.

And the change will come. I've noticed that as long as I'm willing to *be* different, something or someone arrives to show me how. The healthy behavioral pattern you never developed as a child, having been too hurt or traumatized to do so, will be modeled by someone who was *not* hurt as a child in that particular area. Seemingly out of nowhere, he or she will appear in front of you. And slowly but surely, you will learn to behave as you would have wished to behave but were too wounded to know how.

At midlife, the name of the game is change. We're living at a moment of quantum possibility now, not just in terms of our physical age but in terms of the history of the world. It's as though the universe is splitting in two—which perhaps it is. Those who want to continue on the downward course of dysfunction, irresponsibility, entitlement, narcissism, domination, and fear, go here; those who wish to break through to the highest possibility for life on Earth, go there. We can choose to die to who we've been until now, and stand in the light of a new sense of self.

Neither we, nor the world we live in, will go much farther down the road in our current state. We can either let go gracefully of the people we've been, becoming ever more transcendent; or we can let go painfully. Life has a way of making sure we move on. Every moment is an opportunity to exhale old energies and breathe in new life; to exhale fear and inhale love; to exhale littleness and inhale magnitude; to exhale grandiosity and inhale grandeur. Rebirth is a gradual process of giving embrace and welcome to the person we really wish to be.

Take a good look at your life right now. If you don't like something about it, close your eyes and imagine the life you want. Now allow yourself to focus your inner eye on the person you would be if you were living your preferred life. Notice the differences in how you behave and present yourself; allow yourself to spend several seconds breathing in the new image, expanding your energy into this new mold. Hold the image for several seconds and ask God to imprint it on your subconscious mind. Do that every day for 10 minutes or so.

If you share this technique with certain people, the chances are good they'll tell you that it's way too simple. It's up to you what you believe.

Dear God,
Please impress upon me
the vision of whom I am meant to be.
Reveal to me the bigger life
that You would have me live.
Undo the forces that keep me bound
that I might serve You more.
Amen

I THINK MOST OF US HAVE A DREAM, a secret aspiration we never admit to anyone else for fear of being laughed at. Yet the dream remains an image in our head that never really goes away.

At midlife, you start to wonder why that picture has never completely left your mind. It occurs to you that perhaps it's your destiny, planted in your brain like a little yet powerful seedling. You begin to wonder if the dream is still there because you're supposed to live it. Perhaps your subconscious is trying to send you a message about something very important indeed.

At my talks, people often ask, "When am I going to know what I'm supposed to do with my life?" As we age, the question transforms. The only way to know what we should be doing is by focusing on who we should *be*. That doesn't mean there aren't magnificent things we're supposed to do, but God can only work *for* us to the extent that He can work through us. Putting our focus on being who He would have us be is the only sure way we'll ever come close to doing what He would have us do.

Once we've reached a certain age, we tend to recalibrate our expectations. We expect less from the world once we've seen it up close; we know no one is perfect, including ourselves. And that's when we gain an even greater appreciation for the place where perfection does lie. As the grandiosity of the ego diminishes, the grandeur of the spirit is revealed at last. Having truly seen the world, we can see it is tarnished; having finally glimpsed God, we can see He is not. Having seen the juxtaposition between the two is a prerequisite if we're to say to Him, "Please use me; I am Yours."

The part of your life that's over, with all its joy and tears, was spiritual boot camp. It was gestation time for the life that lies ahead of you now. The secret dream you've carried forever, denying its reality even to yourself, has refused to go away and is ready to emerge.

A few times in my life I've heard a voice in my head, speaking as clearly as if a person standing next to me were talking. Once, during a period that I thought was so dark I'd never get over it, I heard these words: "This is not the end. It's the beginning."

And it was.

NEW LIFE EMERGES NOT FROM STRATEGY but from character. Before realizing this, you might think that making plans, devising blueprints for your future or whatever, are the keys to the path ahead. But our real keys to victory are internal. Your state of doing must be matched by the state of your being, or the incongruity will sabotage even your most brilliant plans.

It's been fascinating over the last few years, watching the high and mighty in business and politics fall precipitously—not because their plans didn't work, but because their character flaws undercut those plans. Whether the microphone caught them making racist comments or their greed overcame their common sense, who they were as people made all the difference—more than their résumés, their degrees, or even their past successes. If you fail at the art of being human and staying human, you recklessly court disaster. Yet how do we cultivate the betterment of our humanity? What is the how-to of personal transformation?

What we learn is that the path of right living is walked one moment at a time. Whether you show up for life as a jerk or a saint has little to do with belief or theology; it has to do with personal integrity, and the state of your nervous system at the time. We can be *informed* by abstract belief, but we can't be transformed by it. In *A Course in Miracles*, it says enlightenment begins as abstract theory and takes "a journey without distance from the head to the heart." The heart's transformation is not attained through the mind—it's attained through surrender, authenticity, atonement, forgiveness, faith, honesty, acceptance, vulnerability, humility, willingness, non-judgment, and other characterological values that have to be learned and relearned continuously.

We might skip some lessons at school, but we can't skip any of the lessons of life. They will find us. If a lesson is up for us and we don't learn it now, then it's programmed into the universe that we will just have to learn it later. It's said in *A Course in Miracles* that it's not up to us what we learn, but merely whether we learn through joy or through pain.

But by midlife, we're destined to learn. Whatever parts of you are blocking the emergence of the highest, best you, have simply got to go now. And one way or the other, they will.

Allowing the pain of personal growth to be a crucible of your spirit—the alchemical grail through which the metal of your former self turns into gold—is one of the highest callings of life. Pain can burn you up and destroy you, or burn you up and redeem you. It can deliver you to an entrenched despair, or deliver you to your higher self. At midlife we decide, consciously or unconsciously, the path of the victim or the path of the phoenix when it is rising up at last.

Growth is hard, and laboring a new self can be quite difficult. Growing older just happens; growing wise is something else again. And by a certain point in life, most of us *have* been hurt. We *have* been disappointed. We *have* had dreams die, and might find it hard to forgive ourselves or others. The challenge of age is not to skip life's disappointments but to transcend them. We transcend them by learning the lessons they taught us, however painful, and coming out on the other side prepared to create, with God's help, a new life.

Dear God,
May my spirit be reborn,
that I might be a better person.
I give You my shame
over whom I have sometimes been,
and my hopes for whom I wish to be.
Please receive and transform them both.
Amen

NOT THAT ANY OF THIS IS EASY.

The ego has no intention of allowing us to grow more radiant and spirited as the years go by. It has no intention of allowing us to experience ourselves as fully empowered, joyful, spiritual beings—not if it can help it. Its plan is to destroy that dream—not just by breaking our bodies but by breaking our hearts.

From its headquarters deep in our subconscious minds, the ego magnetizes and manifests our nightmares. It fabricates false testimony to our guilt and guile, finding ways to shame and humiliate us, shape-shifting into insidious forms to taunt and ridicule us at every turn. We're lured into the black hole of self-doubt and self-loathing, as problems both secret and not-so-secret begin to loom on our horizon. With every passing year, we lose courage along with muscle tone.

Yet this is nothing more than the game of life as it must be played by everyone. None of us get to avoid the night, however hard we seek to prolong the day. And the night has its own set of lessons. At a certain point in life, it's simply our destiny to have to face ourselves: to be shown everything not healed within us, challenged to either transform our wounds or to begin to die from them.

If you feel, when looking back on your life so far, that you've wrestled with primal forces and not always won, be assured that you're pretty much like everyone else. It is a rare individual who reaches midlife without a lot to grieve. And whether or not your tears are acknowledged—whether or not you give them the chance to actually fall down your cheeks—there's no question that they're there.

Arrogant in our modernity, we sometimes think we are invulnerable to ancient myths and archetypes. We think we can avoid the descent into the psychic underworld . . . until we realize no one can and no one ever does. And there is a reason for that. The underworld of personal pain and crisis, while difficult, is the inevitable breeding ground for the strengths and talents we were born to embody. It is the psychic birth canal no one can avoid.

Our problems transform themselves into medicine when we learn to face how we created them to begin with. This spiritual medicine—often bitter tasting when it's going down—will one day be seen to have been that which saved your life. From divorce to illness to bankruptcy to whatever other form of loss, you finally come to realize that your crisis was in fact your initiation into the fullness of your self.

Having faced the fire of your initiation and survived its heat, you can now serve others in a whole new way. By being a living testimony to life transformed, you carry in your cells a sacred knowledge, and in your mind and heart a sacred fire. It's not the fire of youth but the fire of Prometheus, who emerged with the light that would light the world. It's a light that you could *only* have gotten from having faced some version of your personal hell, and now you are inoculated to the fires that rage around you. Sometimes only fire can put out fire, and such is the fire that now burns in you. This is not the fire of your destruction but of your victory. It is the fire of your middle years.

Chapter Four

God Only Knows

At a certain point in life, almost everyone is haunted by the ghosts of his or her regrets. There are things we did that we wish we hadn't, and things we didn't do that we wish we had. From family we neglected to friends we abandoned, from ways we acted irresponsibly to opportunities we wasted, situations that seemed unclear to us while we were going through them seem very clear in retrospect.

And during the years when we were carelessly dismissing what we later came to see as the most important things in life, we kept crying out woefully that we were looking for *meaning.* All that time we were starved for meaning, we were lacking it for no other reason than that we weren't *ascribing* meaning to the situations right in front of us! Meaning isn't what a situation gives us; it's what we give to a situation. But who knew?

It's horrifying to recognize we didn't always treat life with the respect it deserved. But at a certain point, facing our shadows is the only way to dispel them. That particular dark night of the soul—facing our self-loathing for the mistakes of our past—is counterintuitively like an entry ticket into a revitalized midlife. Sometimes decades of experience have to be forgiven before we can feel free to move on. Many of us have sent or received letters or made calls expressing things like, "I'm so sorry I hurt you; I was such an idiot fifteen years ago." Regardless of how much discomfort we go through to get there, it's gratifying to feel we've released enough of our past to make room for new growth.

Some people wonder why the energy in their life seems not to be moving forward—when in fact the only thing holding them back is their own unwillingness to face the issues that still need to be faced, the shadows that still need to be owned, and the amends that still need to be made in order to free their energy and restart their engines. As long as we're stuck internally, our lives will be stuck externally; the only way to go wide in life is if we are willing to go deep. It doesn't matter if the problem happened decades ago; the challenge is to face it and deal with it now, so that in the decades ahead you'll be released from the karmic trap of having always to reenact past disasters.

This work is hard to do when we're running around too fast, or wasting our time on electronic speed. Making room in our lives for quiet time is a requirement for spiritual growth; what might appear as a slowing down of our jets is often anything but. A frantic schedule lets us avoid taking a deeper look at ourselves, but by midlife such avoidance simply does not and cannot work anymore. Slower lifestyles, candles and soft music in the house, yoga, meditation, prayer and the like are garden tools that help us regreen. We are focusing on changes that support our deepening. I know a woman who started therapy in her 80s. Her coming to understand so much about her life until this point served more than just herself. It affected conversations with her children that affected their relationships with *their* children, on and on in a never-ending pattern of miracles unleashed by a deeper understanding of herself.

BY MIDLIFE, MOST OF US HAVE a lot of impacted emotional pain. That pain can poison our system or disappear from it. Those are pretty much our only two choices.

Sometimes depression is to the soul what fever is to the body: a way to burn up what needs to be burned up so that health can return. Some dark nights of the soul last months or years, while others just last a night or two. Either way, they're part of a mystical detox of our accumulated fear and despair. Any thought not reconciled with truth remains in our psychic "in-box," put in the trash but not yet deleted from the computer. Whatever energy isn't brought to light, surrendered and transformed, stays in the dark—an insidious force of constant, active attack on both body and soul.

Even if you've lived a pretty good life, unless you've lived it in some isolated mountain village where everyone around you was nice all the time, then you're probably carrying some pain around. In your 30s and 40s you were so busy that you were able to keep distracted, but sometime around your 50s or so, that pain demands to be heard. It *will* be heard. And it's far, far better to hear it in your head and in your soul, than from your doctor when the test results come back and unfortunately they do not look good.

Turning on the TV these days, one feels bombarded by advertisements for sleep medications. It's understandable, of course, that people who have to get up for work the next morning will do anything necessary to get a good night's sleep. But there's a deeper story here, of people seeking help in their efforts to handle the monsters that often emerge from our psyches very late at night. Some of those monsters *need* to be let out. They need to be freed from the caves they live in. They bring messages of pain, it's true, and yet the pain they bring is often important pain. If you don't feel the guilt, how will you ever reach your motivation to make amends? If you don't feel the self-loathing, how will you ever reach the motivation to act more responsibly next time? If you avoid the pain, you'll miss the gain. Just suppressing the monsters only makes them larger. Allowing them out—and allowing yourself to finally face them—is the only way to make sure that they will ever go away.

It's not always fun to face your past—not the whitewashed, historically revised version, but the real backstory you don't look at daily because it would make you so unhappy if you did. And the actual events probably weren't any worse than what others have been through in their lives. Compared to other people, you might not have even done so badly. But wherever you didn't live up to your personal best, shame remains like an underground toxin. You live with regrets that haunt you, perhaps rarely during the day when the ego's delusional worldview holds sway, but during those nights when no pill or drink or amount of sex can keep them from you. They move through locked doors in your mind as though they're ghosts, which they are. And no amount of "Go on now, go!" can shoo them away.

Only the rigorous work of taking a fearless moral inventory will do that—the bravery to respect your conscience, to know that if something's up for review then it's best to review it. In the words of the ancient Greek playwright Aeschylus, "He who learns must suffer. And even in our sleep pain that cannot forget falls drop by drop upon the heart, and in our own despair, against our will, comes wisdom to us by the awful grace of God." Numbing ourselves—while sleeping or waking—will not erase the pain; only forgiveness and love can do that. Then, through the power of atonement and grace, the ghosts will go back to the nothingness whence they came. And they will be no more. The past is over, and you are free.

Dear God,
Please forgive me the
mistakes in my past.
May neither I
nor anyone else
be bound by them.
Please God,
may I begin again.
The past is over.
May it touch me not.
Amen

One of the most pernicious of the ego's taunts at midlife is the nagging fear that we're running out of time. Yet time expands when our consciousness does. Our enemy is not really time, but our *false thinking* about time.

In the Bible it states: "And time shall be no more," but rather than foreshadowing the end of the world, this indicates the end of our experiencing time the way that we do now. Midlife slows down when we live it well. In fact, we have more time than we thought. The key to stretching time is to go deeper into the present. When we do, we find something wonderful there: choices we didn't realize we had in the days when we were moving too fast to see them.

By a certain point, most of us have experienced enough of the world to no longer be naïve about it. We know what it gives and we know what it takes away. We have memories of joy and we have memories of sorrow. Our challenge, in both cases, is to not dwell in the memories of pain.

As long as there's life, there's the possibility of love. And where there is love, there is always hope. No matter what the mirror says, no matter what your doctor says, no matter what the establishment says—there is hope. It's tempting to feel at times that you blew it in the past and there's nothing you can do to redeem yourself. Or that the cruelty of the world defeated you and you can't rise back up. But the miracle of midlife is that nothing that happened before this moment has any bearing on what's possible now, except that what you learned from it can be fuel for a magnificent future.

Miracles are available in any moment when we bring the best of ourselves forward. It isn't the amount of your years that will determine the life you live now, but the amount of your love. Our future isn't determined by anything that happened 20 years ago, 30 years ago, or even 10 minutes ago. It's determined by who we are and what we think, right here, right now, in this instant. Almost every hour of every day, we'll find ourselves in a situation where we can be now who we weren't before, because we *know* now what we didn't know before. And from this newness in our being springs fresh opportunities we could never have imagined. God specializes in new beginnings.

I had an experience once that depressed me greatly. I felt wounded by something in my past and fairly hopeless about my future. Around that time, I moved into a house on the water, where I had a view of the sunrise each day more gorgeous than anything I had ever seen. Every morning's sky looked like a Japanese woodcut that had come to life, with black branches slowly turning deep green, ebony sky turning hot pink on top of the branches, and a beautiful bright turquoise below. I had never experienced nature as such a deeply spiritual thing before. It was so extraordinary. I felt I'd been led to that house, and to that bedroom view, as part of my healing.

Every day my eyes would automatically open as the sun began to rise. I'd lie there and not just look at the dawn; the dawn would *enter* me. The imprint of sunrise—of a new day following the darkness of night—made its way into my cells. And one morning it was as though I heard the voice of God, telling me as I witnessed the dawn that "Such is the work I will do within you." I too would experience a new dawn after the dark night of my soul. God would give me a new beginning. I knew it then. And as I closed my eyes and drifted back to sleep, I thanked Him with all my heart. And in time, my heart was healed.

I'M OFTEN AMAZED when watching Olympic ice-skaters. Someone who has practiced something thousands, literally thousands, of times, gets in front of a worldwide TV audience in the most important competition of their lives, and makes a fall that could ruin all their dreams in one split second. How many of us would just completely fall apart at that point? But not them. They keep going. They've got another triple axel to do 1.2 seconds later. They simply cannot allow their future to be determined by the past. And that's not just a physical skill. It's an emotional skill, a psychological discipline. It's an expertise that anyone who wants to progress into a prosperous, creative, and exciting second half of life needs to develop.

It's not simply that "what's past is past." It's bigger, somehow holier than that. It's that what has happened until now was a set of lessons—often extraordinary, often painful. Yet all that was ever going on was that you were being given the chance to become the person you're capable of being. Some lessons you passed, and some you failed and will have to take again. Some you enjoyed, and some you resisted and might have hated. But they've left you a better person, a more humble person, a more available person, a more vulnerable person, a wiser person, a more noble person. And that is your redemption. From that, all things are possible. A youthful body is wonderful, but it's not all it's cracked up to be when you're not yet who you were born to be. And once you are, the cracks in your body can have a beauty of their own. You don't have to be young to be fabulous.

Yet how do we do emotionally what those ice-skaters do physically? How do we get up again when life has thrown us down? How do we get over the past?

Without forgiveness, it cannot be done.

One night I was lying in bed, nearing sleep, and I realized I'd been taken to some dimension I'd never experienced before. I say "taken" because it just seemed to happen. In this place I knew I was older, and I knew I couldn't have entered the space if I were not. There was a light, a luminescence that was clearly something

I couldn't have known until this point. I knew then that if I could live in this place on a consistent basis, I would never see it as a lesser world. It wasn't a booby prize; it was clearly a reward. It wasn't as though I was carrying baggage; it was as though I had received a gift.

"Oh, this is what age is!" I said to myself, relieved that it was so wonderful. But a response came clearly: "Well, not for everyone." I was visiting an inner domain that was not a given. It had to be chosen. It was revealed to me in one of those momentary gifts of grace, perhaps, but only as an enticement, a demonstration of what was mine to earn. Before the present could start to shine like that, I would have to learn how to forgive.

It's fairly easy staying loving and serene when others always act the way you want them to, but that's not a realistic picture of life. Everyone's imperfect, everyone's wounded, and most of us have been somewhat scathed at one time or another by the casual cruelty of others.

Forgiveness involves faith in a love that's greater than hatred. It's willingness to see the light in someone's soul even when their personality has harbored darkness. Forgiveness doesn't mean that someone didn't act horribly; it simply means that we choose not to focus on their guilt. In focusing on guilt, we make it real to us, and in making it real to us, we make it real *for* us. The only way to deliver ourselves from vulnerability to other people's transgressions is by identifying with the part of them that lies beyond their behavior. We can look beyond someone's mistakes to the innocence in their souls. Doing so, we not only free *them* from the weight of our condemnation, but we free ourselves as well.

That is the miracle of forgiveness.

Forgiveness isn't just about being *nice*—it's about being spiritually intelligent. We can have a grievance or we can have a miracle, but we cannot have both. We can build a case against someone, or we can be happy. Any justification I come up with for an attack on another person is just my ego's ploy to keep *me* in pain. To the extent that I identify with what you did to me, I will be at the effect of what you did to me. The only way I can free myself is if I am willing to free you.

A concept it has taken me years to embrace fully is that I am 100 percent responsible for my own life. 100 percent responsible doesn't mean 34 percent responsible, and it doesn't mean 96 percent responsible. Unless you're willing to accept that you're *100* percent responsible for your own experience, then you can't call forth your best life.

Some people nurse grievances that go back 20 years. At a certain point, however, it becomes harder to blame all your problems on what someone did to you that long ago. No matter what they did, the real culprit is the one who's let 20 years pass without getting over it.

BY MIDLIFE, MOST PEOPLE CARRY AROUND a bag full of painful memories and cringe moments we wish we could forget. Like a plane before take-off, we can't ascend to the next level of things without getting rid of all that emotional weight. Then the question becomes, how do we do that? In the final analysis there is really only one way: to forgive it. Some awful things might have happened to us during the years leading up to this moment, but we are still responsible for how we choose to interpret them. And that's what forgiveness is: a reinterpretation of events, releasing us from the burden of memories that otherwise will continue to weigh us down. Whether or not we choose to forgive the past determines whether it will uplift us or emotionally sink us.

Yes, there may have been some people who viciously wronged you. But it serves you to realize any ways you might have made it easy for them to do it. Atoning for our own mistakes is as important as forgiving other people for theirs. In *A Course in Miracles*, it says we pay a very high price for not taking 100 percent responsibility for our lives. The price is that we won't be able to change it. As easy as it is to blame others for what went wrong in our lives, that brutally honest look in the mirror—while it might hurt temporarily—is far more liberating. The challenge of midlife is to start over, and it can't be done unless we do that work. It's not that forgiveness is always easy. But it's imperative.

My friend Gina went through a terrible divorce, giving her plenty of opportunity to choose between forgiveness and blame. After 11 years of what she had thought was a good marriage—what anyone who'd ever seen them together assumed was a great marriage—her husband wanted out. I've never seen a relationship that was all one person's issues, so I'm making no judgment here on either person's behavior. But I can say from having walked alongside her that her path was the path of forgiveness . . . and it paid off. Did she go through a year of hell? Yes, she did. But her consistent efforts to bless and forgive her ex-husband—a man whom she refused to cast out of her heart although he seemed to have cast her out of his—was not only inspiring to witness, but demonstrative of the way that forgiveness works miracles. She continued to lay claim to the love between them, regardless of the fact that the form of the relationship was being torn apart. She was hurt, but not bitter. She continued to have faith. He could leave the marriage, but she would not give up on the love between them. And within 18 months, they'd swung full circle. They were no longer married but the friendship survived.

That was important for Gina, not just so she could be at peace with her past marriage but so she could be at peace with any man she met afterward. If bitterness in our past is brought into the present, it then sabotages our future. Even in the midst of her divorce, my daughter and I would joke that Gina was a man magnet. And we could understand why. Allowing herself to feel her pain without defending against it, she grew suppler instead of tougher. She didn't harden at the loss of love, the way some people do. I watched her mature, but I never saw her harden. And love kept rushing in.

You can live the rest of your life reacting to and replaying what went before, but that won't serve you or deliver you to the shining place. And everyone you meet will subconsciously know how you've responded to your past. They will know whether you're stuck there or better for having been there. "Forgive and forget" is not mere platitude. Many say, "Yes, I do forgive, but I will never forget." Beware that sentiment, for it leaves you subtly in the thrall of suffering. Do forget what was done to you; just remember the lessons you learned from it. Drop the cross. Embrace the sky.

Dear God,
Please teach me
how to forgive.
Show me the innocence in others,
and the innocence in myself.
I surrender to You
my judgmental thoughts.
May I see beyond them
to the gentle peace
that only forgiveness brings.
Amen

THE FEAR-BASED EGO gathers evidence at every turn, making forgiveness hard. The ego is obsessed with two big cases: one against everybody else, and one against you.

Sometimes the face at the center of your bull's-eye doesn't belong to anyone else. Yours is the name on the docket of the case you feel compelled to prosecute—you, for your past errors; you, for your past stupidity; you, for your past immaturity; you, for your past irresponsibility; you, for just being you.

Prosecutorial witnesses are everywhere, and the courtroom is in your head. The ego is not on a search for justice but for guilt, for that is what it feeds on. Its case against you is not just based on the notion that you did something wrong, but that in some fundamental way you *are* wrong. That's a hard rap to beat. Who could ever sleep well if convinced that everything about them is just *wrong?*

You feel you've blown it on so many levels, in so many ways, and on some nights for whatever reason it all comes back so clearly. . . . What a lovely life, having 20-year-old bad memories shooting through your brain like bazookas from hell—which, in a way, they are. And you have nowhere to put them except in that big fat file called "All the Ways I Screwed Up." How can you feel that there's goodness ahead when you feel that in the past you have been so bad? How can you have much hope for the future when your take on the past is so relentlessly vicious? And how can you really defend yourself against a ruthless prosecutor who is an aspect of yourself?

You know the religious image of "burning in hell forever"? Well, now you know what it means: anxiety and guilt and self-hatred without end. It wasn't God who sent you there, but rather the enemy in your own mind. The ego, the fear-based self, the shadow—whatever name you choose to call it—is on active patrol to burn down your peace of mind.

The reason for faith that you can and will escape those flames is that God guarantees your fundamental innocence. He created you innocent, and what He creates is changeless and indestructible. Have you made mistakes? Who hasn't? But God's will is to correct our mistakes, not punish us for them. We are punished *by* our sins, not for them. It's the ego that both sets us up to do the wrong thing and then punishes us savagely for having done so.

An all-merciful God has already dismissed every case against you before the ego has a chance to mount it. Your mistakes, no matter how bad you might think they were, did not emanate from your self as He created you. That's why remembering who you truly are is the key to deliverance from the flames of self-condemnation.

You're no better or worse than anyone else. No matter how much you might regret your past, there's someone out there who regrets his or hers more. The path to happiness is not determined by whether or not we made mistakes in the past. What paves the way to happiness is whether or not we turn our mistakes into catalysts for personal growth and illumination.

Think of everything you've ever been through, and try to reinterpret it gently. All the love you ever gave was real. All the love anyone ever gave you was real. Everything else was simply an illusion, no matter how bitter or cruel it might have been in your experience.

I'm not going to insult you by saying, "Just forgive yourself." God forgives you, because He never saw you as anything but innocent. Your mistakes did not change the ultimate truth about you or alter the permanent nature of God's universe. Your ego is not that powerful. Truly atone for your errors, make amends where possible, and you'll be free to begin again.

According to *A Course in Miracles,* in the moments when you were not your best self—when you didn't stand up as the most loving you could be—then all the good you deflected is being held in trust for you until you're ready to receive it. God will return to you the years that the locusts have eaten. And the past as you know it shall be no more.

Wherever there was fear, love will ultimately prevail. Whether in response to your own mistakes or to the cruelty of the world, God will always have the final say. And His say will always be how very much that you are loved.

Dear God,
Please help me to forgive myself
for what I did and did not do.
Pour forth upon me
Your infinite mercy,
that my life might be redeemed.
Take away my shame, dear God,
and heal my broken heart.
Amen

WHENEVER I FEEL AT THE EFFECT of my past, I try to remember people whose experiences have been not only worse than mine but worse than any I could even imagine. And yet they rose above.

My friend Naomi Warren was a Holocaust survivor of three Nazi concentration camps during World War 2. The war began on her 19th birthday, as German troops crossed the Polish border on September 1, 1939. Living in Warsaw at the time, she went from enjoying the life of a young woman preparing to go to college in England to hiding from the Nazis with her mother, husband, brother, and sister-in-law. Her father had already been arrested by the Russians and sent to Siberia. In 1943, having survived the bombing of Warsaw, Naomi and the other members of her family were huddled into a cattle car for a horrendous trip that many didn't survive, and taken to a concentration camp at Auschwitz.

She was at Auschwitz from the age of 22 to 24. My problems at that age? Romance, career, and the like. Hers? Adolf Hitler.

Naomi's husband, mother, and sister-in-law all died at Auschwitz. Her mother died in a crematorium; then her sister-in-law, having told Naomi one morning that she simply would not go to work that day ("I cannot stand it," she said. "I cannot live like this.") disappeared and never returned. My friend and millions of others lived in Nazi concentration camps under conditions as horrifying as any forced on human beings by other human beings before or since.

Ultimately, Naomi survived the war. After emigrating to the United States in 1946, she married and was widowed a second time, leaving her with three young children to raise as a single mother. If anyone might have been given a pass, forgiven for just giving up, it would have been Naomi. Yet that simply isn't who she was. Her character was bigger than her circumstances. She raised her children beautifully, started an import-export company that eventually became phenomenally successful (at a time when not many women were doing that, by the way), and lived through the years as an inspiration to countless who have known her—including myself.

In 2002, Naomi went back to Germany with her son. As their plane approached Berlin and she sat looking out the window at the land below, he asked how she was feeling. Her response, she said, surprised even her: "It's very strange, but I feel good about this. I am here on my own terms. I am not being brought here by anybody. I am coming of my own free will."

Visiting Wannsee—where in 1942 Hitler and his top aides made plans for "the final solution," or complete extermination of the Jews—Naomi collapsed. Yet her reconciliation with her past continued. In 2003, she made an emotional journey back to Auschwitz. After having cried the entire way there, she had a strange experience once she arrived. Upon entering the gate with its famously ironic inscription, "Arbeit macht frei" ("Work makes you free"), she felt herself becoming very, very strong. She didn't feel the pain she'd expected. Rather, she said she felt a spirit of victory move through her as she realized: "Oh my goodness, I've come back—and I survived! I came here to perish, but I did not! He who wanted to destroy me was himself destroyed, but I survived. I am a survivor!" In that moment, she knew what it meant to *be* a survivor—not only physically, but emotionally and spiritually as well. And she was free.

"I felt I could build on my past," she has said, "but I knew I could not live in it. In spite of the fact that I lived through the Holocaust, I have never dwelled on it. I went through something so terrible, but I like to think something good can come from it. I have so much more empathy. I like to think I'm a better person because of it.

"Hope is always in us. In spite of the fact that everything looks so bleak, there's something in all of us that keeps thinking things are going to get better. I knew I had to look to the future. I had to always ask what I could do *now* to be more productive. I wanted to live for the future, for myself and for my children. And I did."

Naomi once said to me, "As I walked out of Auschwitz for the last time, I said to myself, 'Hitler got two years of my life. He will not get another day.'"

Times are tough for many people right now. But if my friend Naomi could rebuild her life after what she went through, who among us doesn't have in deep reserve the strength it might take to rebuild ours? We have a moral responsibility—not only to ourselves but to a rising tide of collective hope—to do everything possible to rise up from whatever ashes might litter our past. Yesterday was yesterday and yesterday is over. Today is today and tomorrow stands in front of us. What we do with it is up to us.

What happened to you yesterday might not have been wonderful or even under your control. But who you become because of it, or in spite of it, is completely up to you. I've known people who lived through a fraction of the trauma that Naomi Warren lived through, yet stayed in the muck of their grievances and victimization for decades. What her story demonstrates is that we are not our past. It's not what life threw at us that determines what our life will be now; the future is determined by how much of ourselves we're willing to throw into life.

My friend Naomi passed from this world at the age of 96, but she remains a beacon of light to everyone who knew her. She told me once that she saw herself not as a victim, but as a victor. If Naomi could move on after

Auschwitz, then who among us for whatever reason can claim we cannot move on?

Dear God,
Please take away from me
the pain of my past.
Remove the arrows
that have pierced my heart,
and heal my open wounds.
No matter what happened to me then,
May it make me a better person now.
Amen

Chapter Five

Women of a Certain Age

I always intuited that when I was in my 50s, I would allow myself to stop hiding. I found the world so frightening when I was younger, so unexplainable or perhaps just unexplained to *me,* that I struggled to cope by trying to hide. Some would look at my career and say, "I would hardly call that hiding," but no one knows what other people might be holding inside and not allowing themselves to express.

I experienced a peculiarly American split, a neurotic affliction that women of my generation were particularly prey to. I didn't realize it consciously—few of us did—but the message we internalized in the name of liberation was that we could only be liberated if we became like men. We could be hot and sexy, or we could be smart and taken seriously; we could not be both. So many of us did what we thought we had to do: We suppressed the goddess, the wild wise woman, in order to make it in a world that we'd subconsciously joined in its disdain for the essentially female.

I don't think I fully enjoyed being a woman, without any sense of shame, until I was well into my 40s. Before that, I was ambivalent about it. And my ambivalence about the juicier aspects of being female attracted ambivalence in men and women alike. If we feel guilty about something, whether we deserve the attack on ourselves or not, we'll attract someone into our lives to reflect and articulate our self-condemnation. Whatever I've done in my life—no matter how outrageous—if I thought it was okay, then so did most of the people around me. But when I've been unclear or ashamed of something, then there's always been someone there to take an emotional bludgeon to my heart. One of the gifts of age is that it finally becomes easier to ignore other people's opinions. We've been through enough to know our own true feelings, and we're ready to live the lives we would have lived all along if we had thought it was okay.

I was the classic Jungian "father's daughter" subconsciously—or maybe not subconsciously—mimicking my father's life while under the wrong impression that my mother's wasn't "important" enough. The emotional price I paid for what I now see to have been some delusion of masculine superiority was tremendous. My mother knew things—wise, earthy things—that she tried to tell me, but I wouldn't hear.

Once I was sitting around with girlfriends discussing an unmarried friend's choice of whether to have an abortion. All of a sudden, my mother chimed in, "Aren't you girls old enough to know there's no such thing as an illegitimate child?" We told her there was a question about paternity. She bristled. "Do you girls think that every person you knew growing up had a daddy who was *really* their daddy? In *my* day, women knew how to keep their *mouths shut!*" We were stunned, silenced. A woman who we assumed didn't know as much as we did in fact knew so much more—about the facts, and about being human.

Now it makes me proud to think that I'm my father's daughter; but I'm my mother's daughter too. Women entering midlife today don't have the same hang ups we had when I was their age, because time moves on. But just as every generation has its own wisdom, every generation has its own challenges as well. The important thing is to face those challenges, to be honest with ourselves about them, to bring them up for review both within our hearts and among our friends. What am I missing? What am I disowning? What am I not appreciating? What am I unwilling to become?

Midlife is a path we must forge consciously, or it will unfold according to the unconscious dictates of fear instead of love. Most women today, even in the most advanced societies, begin to feel the emotional undertows of ageism and misogyny as midlife comes upon us. Embracing the ancient truths of feminine power that lie within us all, often buried, as they are in our modern age, we begin to claim the awesome forces that lie latent within. We aren't nearly so vulnerable to the lies of the world when the truth of the heart rests firmly in our awareness. It's an awareness that came through our mothers, and through theirs, through theirs, and through theirs. We should thank them. Being young has nothing on being aware, at last, that there is a crown above us all.

Dear God,
To whatever extent
I fail to respect
the power and glory
of the female sex,
may my mind be corrected
and my heart be transformed.
Reveal to me the feminine truths
That are divine and live within me.
Amen

IN ANY ADVANCED MAMMALIAN SPECIES that survives and thrives, there's a common characteristic: The adult female of the species displays fierce behavior when she senses a threat to her young. Lionesses and tigresses grow fierce when they detect danger to their offspring. Among hyenas, hardly known as the most tender of creatures, the adult females encircle their cubs while they're feeding, keeping adult males at bay until the babies have been fed.

You'd think that we would do better than the hyenas. Yet there are reasons why we don't, and why we haven't. Women in our part of the world haven't been held back by a lack of political power—not for almost a hundred years—but by centuries-old forces of misogynistic prejudice. Emotional chains are still chains that bind. We stopped burning witches, but we still haven't completely routed out of Western consciousness our suspicion of the powerful female.

During the Middle Ages, the word *witch* meant "wise woman"; the projection of "ugliness" onto witches was simply a caricature fabricated by the early church in its intent to denigrate and suppress female power. Our earthiness as well as our spirituality was deemed an enemy. Where pagan priestesses initiated men into their manhood through sexual rites, Christianity would declare our sexuality holy only if used for procreation.

A woman who could no longer make babies, then, had no "holy" function left. Indeed, during the witch burnings, older unmarried women were usually the first to die. If you weren't cavorting with the church and its teachings, you were deemed to be cavorting with the devil. And while the notion is ridiculous, there's nothing humorous about several hundred thousand or more women burning at the stake. The witch burnings were a female holocaust.

Women have been *afraid* to show our fierceness—on behalf of our children, our planet, or anything else—because we haven't wanted to be labeled "witches." The fact that the consonant has been changed from "w" to "b" has not changed the emotional reality for us. We don't want to be seen as "bitchy," "angry," "strident." I know from experience how modern witch burning works today. I know the fire, and I know the pain. I understand the cellular memory, and the modern fear too many women feel—"If they're mocking Marianne and I show up to support her, then they might mock me too." It makes all the sense in the world why women too often grow silent about things that matter most.

Pagan women exalted the divine connection between an individual person and the natural world. Their priestesses ritualistically connected souls to each other and to the world around them. Their destruction at the hands of the early church was a tragedy not only for them, but also for the development of Western civilization. For their disappearance in many ways presaged today's environmental crisis, paving the way for an era in which it has been deemed acceptable for humanity to dominate nature. In order to end this global crisis, we must dismantle the thought-forms that produced it. Part of our atonement for how we have desecrated the earth involves atonement for how we desecrated a culture in which the wisdom of women was given its true due.

I wish I could say that all of that was over but it's not. And not only in parts of the world where women are still stoned to death for suspected adultery, or murdered for not wearing a veil, or denied an education or even the right to sing or even speak in public. Even in the United States, there are political forces at work right now making every effort to deny women rights that we thought we could take for granted. Not only women's rights, but even women's lives are at stake. Women of all ages must carry the torch of enlightened understanding at what is now a darkened hour.

Midlife is a time to assume leadership—whether in our families, business, communities, or politics. Not because we finally know all the answers—hardly! But because we finally know what meaningful questions need to be asked. It's not questions like, "How will that serve the financial bottom line?" It's questions like, "How will that affect the earth, the children, the future of the human race?"

A friend once told me, "Fifty is the age past which you don't care what other people think anymore." At midlife we must no longer disown our truth, or our power. Fortified by conviction gained over many chapters lived, having failed at some things and succeeded at others, we are prepared to lead the way in the creation of a better world. Life has prepared us for the role. We don't feel the need any longer to ask anyone for permission. You arrive at the time of your life when you will give *yourself* permission to live a more significant life.

We are remembering at last our forgotten powers, no longer to physically procreate, perhaps, but to spiritually regenerate. We're going to change history; we're going to turn the *Titanic* around this time before it hits the iceberg; we're going to miraculously stop the insane, suicidal march now presided over by the governments of the world; and it's going to happen *because we say so.*

Women must reclaim the ecstatic feminine impulse before we can appear again in the fullness of our glory. The witches of yesterday will rest, I hope, having found across the ages in a new generation of women the pity and compassion they deserve. We grieve for them and for ourselves. For every woman who cannot find her voice or attract her love or express her power or heal our world, there was a woman burned alive for trying to do so. As we unearth our long-buried passion for female self-actualization, let us never forget the price paid by so many for making the effort. May they, our dear dishonored sisters, find peace.

As a little girl, I remember being drawn to girls a few years older than me. I felt the same when I was 30 and 40, and I feel that way today. I've always felt that those who walked life's path just a few years ahead of me had something important to show me.

Now I see the pattern from the other side: I have younger friends who feel to me, and I think to them as well, like my spiritual younger siblings. They're growing into their power and show me the honor of valuing mine. It's a very important role in life, doing everything we can to model our best selves to those who are younger. It doesn't mean more years have made us perfect. Hardly. But it does mean that we take very seriously now the effort to live as responsibly as we can. There's something sort of unseemly about a woman who ages but refuses to grow up.

Mentoring isn't just something nice you do, or even necessarily a conscious choice. It's a pattern you magnetize to yourself as part of the natural order. As you yourself grow more mature, those behind you in time—ones who would be most served by your teaching—automatically appear in your life. And by teaching, I mean not only what you know but what you demonstrate.

I can't imagine where I'd be today had there not been those who arrived on my path to show me what I needed to see at just the moment when I needed to see it. And they still do. Now it's also my turn to try to help put together some piece of life's puzzle for those who see me as one who's done it herself. How we behave, how we do or do not seek to bring harmony to the world around us, reflect energy we're beaming out to those around us all the time. A younger friend who is like a little sister to me has said to me more than once, "You think I'm ignoring you, but I am listening to every word."

Sometimes I meet younger people at my lectures who remind me of something I wrote in a book or said in a talk. I know the thrill of being young and hearing ideas you haven't heard before, seeing someone model a role in the culture that you feel beckoning to you. I was there once. And now I'm here. I meet the young woman telling me she wants to someday do what I do; I smile and say, "Then do it!" I remember the young man who handed me a rose; I received with gratitude his generosity and respect.

The elders are honored when we behave more honorably. The younger you are the more you know certain things, and the older you are the more you know other things. A beautiful intergenerational dance begins as we reach midlife. People aren't looking to us for quite the same things that they used to, and the gifts we give them aren't quite the same either. You start to see that age is a mystery, a constant ebb and flow of wisdom we're learning and other wisdom we're dispensing. Entering a new stage, we find there are things that begin to fall away. But new life only begins to blossom when we're ready to let them go.

Dear God,
Help me to release the things
that are no longer mine.
May I be worthy
of an honored role
in the lives of those
behind me.
Show me how
to use Your gifts,
and how to pass them on.
Amen

I'VE HEARD MYTHICAL and not-so-mythical stories of older women who moved into a convent, as though their worldly ride was over and from here on out they would drop the veil on worldly concerns. But I've come to think that the convent experience is an inner domain, maybe externalized and maybe not. The convent that matters is a space in the heart where you live for God—we can't live for God if we're not living for one another. You live for God not as an escape from the world but as an effort to live in it with greater compassion. We free ourselves from obsessive goals of achieving this or manifesting that, making our highest to live a more impeccable life.

When I used to think of women in the Middle Ages going into a convent at middle age (that probably would have meant 30 or 35!), I felt so sorry for them. No fun. No excitement. No sex. And Lord, what boring bedrooms! But today the convent experience—the internal variety—means anything but that. It means no fun that isn't laced with the sacred, no excitement that isn't laced with the sacred, no sex that isn't laced with the sacred. The sacred means that which binds us to God, and because we are one with God, it binds us to ourself. The fun doesn't stop when we come to understand that; only the *neurosis* stops when we understand it. Freud defined neurosis as "separation from self." A sacred experience means one we enter into with the truth of who we are, whether it's singing a song or holding a child or starting a project or trying to change the world.

When I was young I didn't know how to celebrate life, though in retrospect there was so much to celebrate. At midlife I realized it was my responsibility to mark the fabulousness of life, not only in the big things but in the little ones. To not take so much for granted. For what we appreciate appreciates. When we make a big deal about life, life makes a big deal about us. If God were leaving us a text, I think it would say: "Enjoy yourself."

I once read an interview with actress Cameron Diaz where she said that she didn't think being light and bubbly was any less valid than being dark and moody. I took that in for a moment, realizing it had taken me decades longer to see this than it had taken her. Women in my generation wanted to be taken so *seriously,* primarily because our mothers weren't. We suppressed our joy under the false assumption that joy is silly in some way. In fact, it's when you realize how serious life is that you take yourself *less* seriously, and take every opportunity to laugh when it comes along. I once read where Mariane Pearl, the widow of slain *Wall Street Journal* reporter Daniel Pearl, has said that happiness is an act of resistance.

And happiness can be created from almost anything if we're willing to engage with life. A close friend who is now in her eighth decade has, among other artistic attributes, a phenomenal sense of fashion. She is one of those fashionistas that lights up the Internet, and any room she enters. She has an amazing knack for finding things that are basically priceless, that are for sale somewhere for practically nothing. And she turns them into art. Her life is a creative process, and there is no way you can encounter her and not start to smile. I'm always saying to her, "How did you doooooo that?!" Particularly as we age, we're so tempted to say about so many things, "Oh I can't do that anymore." But that's just a thought. The spirit has no age, and no lack of creative potential.

Flowers don't apologize for being beautiful, and neither should we. Our beauty changes as we age, but it needed disappear. It has occurred to me that I've never seen a statue of a Greek or Hindu goddess in which she wasn't dressed to the nines. The idea that a *spiritual* woman chooses to have less going on for her in the looks department was introduced into our thought system by a woman-hating institution, remember—the same club that used to burn women at the stake. So when anyone suggests a woman should dress plainly and simply in order to show her piety, I rush to put on a camisole. Makeup and jewelry go back longer than *they* do; thousands of years ago, women wore rouge and rubies and knew exactly what they were doing. Queen Esther didn't save her people by looking unattractive that night. Any effort to desexualize women is an effort to disempower us; making us feel guilty about wanting to look good is more of the same oppressive game that would have us hide other aspects of our power as well.

Our society is of two minds about a mature woman trying to look good. She's shamed for "letting herself go," or she's shamed for trying to hold it together. All this talk about "natural aging" is sort of ridiculous, given that pesticides, pollution, carcinogens, the hole in the ozone, worry, economic anxiety, and divorce statistics aren't exactly natural forces. There's nothing necessarily *natural* about all that stress on your face. If a woman wants to order the newest online product, get filler, or employ any other cosmetic procedure, then if it makes her happy she should do it. I don't see aging with a regimen for staying hot and happening as any less *graceful* than simply appreciating your wrinkles.

It's not "serious" to want to look good? What's so serious about *not* looking good? The late seriously gorgeous and ageless Gloria Vanderbilt once said that beauty is a gift from God, which we have a responsibility to care for as long as we can. A woman taking care of herself—both in body and in spirit—is part of her participation in a wild and wonderful female adventure. That adventure is emotional, intellectual, spiritual, and sexual. Limits to our beauty exist more in our mind than anywhere else.

I've known people that society today would call "old" who had more going on in the sex department than some of the younger people I've known. Desexualizing ourselves, or allowing society to desexualize us, is a blow to our spiritual power. Let's remember that the ancient world was dotted with romantic and erotic temples.

We should honor our function as keepers of the erotic flame. The bedroom is where we both conceive our children, repair our lovers and heal ourselves, all of which fuel the regeneration of the human race.

Yet whether our energy expresses itself sexually or not, it's magical and important. The truth is, nature helps us when we're younger—the glowing skin, the firm butt, the perky breasts are all reflections of nature's intention that the chances for sex are maximized and the species will survive. That's great for the young ones, but once we've completed our childbearing years nature doesn't really *care* whether or not we ever have sex! We're not getting help from nature the way we used to. We can't just wake up, throw on jeans, and know it takes very little else to have it going on. We don't get looked at the way we used to. We lose that power in a room that most younger women have just by walking into it. It's ridiculous to pretend we don't feel the change. Of course we do. It's one of the things we have to grieve as we enter midlife. In today's world we might still look great—and for a long time—but the voluptuousness of youth is like a sun that shines and then it sets. Another kind of power replaces it, but it's a transition that doesn't come quickly.

We lose our youth, but we don't have to lose our magic. Sexual magic isn't only about babies; it's about enchantment. We don't lure a partner into bed only to procreate; we lure them into bed in order to set their hearts on fire. We share a bewitched and bewitching space so that a romantic alchemy can deliver us both to a higher place. This isn't a joy that stops when we age; in a way, it's a job we don't *understand* 'til we age. Midlife is *not* the time to disenchant ourselves, sexually or in any other way. If anything, it's a time to turn our magic in full force.

EXCITEMENT DOESN'T KNOCK AT OUR DOOR any less when we're older than when we're younger; the difference is that when we're younger, we were more likely to let it in. With age, we start growing *ambivalent* about excitement. We might say that we want it, but at the same time we start to block it. We remember too many things that didn't work out, so maybe we shouldn't try. Or we're not sure you have the energy for it. A surefire way to diminish our energy is to start saying no in places where we used to more often say yes.

My father lived to be 85, and he was exciting his entire life. He used to always say, "You've gotta have a sense of adventure!" And boy did he. It wasn't just evidenced by his dramatic adventures traveling the world; it was evidenced by his approach to everyday life. The way he rode in a convertible even when it was raining because "Only sissies put the top up." The way he taught his small children Stanislavsky acting exercises as a substitute for normal games. The way he wore a Greek sailor's cap around, although we lived in Texas, just in case the Greek navy might call and say they needed him! My father was like a male version of Auntie Mame. Whatever he did, he was *into* it—fully, passionately, and with total vigor. A man like my father wasn't looking to vitamins to give him more energy. He looked to *life* to give him more energy, by giving it so much of his own.

In the Russian Orthodox Church, there is the concept of the "passion bearer." I think that's what midlife makes us: the passion bearers of life, people who have been through enough to have felt the passion of life's pain as well as its triumphs. To whatever extent we find joy in our own becoming, we help others find joy in theirs.

In ancient cultures, it was the role of the elder to lead tribal celebrations. Why? Because we're the holders of the excitement factor. When a woman 20 years younger than I am announces that she's pregnant, I feel I'm fulfilling some primal function by letting her know I think it's the most exciting thing in the world. It's as though I'm representing the opinion of something larger than myself. A teenager gets on a sports team or enters an essay-writing contest; a young woman gets into the managerial training program at the company she's been working at for years; a young man starts his own company or makes his first business deal—in every case, an older person's enthusiasm could be a memory someone holds for a lifetime. People need to know that the world is on their side, and for a younger person, the "world" is often represented by whatever adult he or she is speaking to at the time.

Celebration isn't passive; it's an active energy mover. I've heard young people denigrate something I know in their hearts represents a dream come true, saying something like, "Oh, it's not that big a deal." But if I say with determination, "Oh, *yes* it is!" then their entire attitude shifts.

I do this for them, and I do it for myself. Once you've lived enough and cried enough tears of your own, you know how blessed it is to have something to smile about. People who are passionate about life don't have a positive attitude because they don't know any better. They're often positive because they *do* know better. They know that heartbreak could happen any day. If it's not happening today, let's give thanks.

I used to have a bottle of good champagne in my refrigerator. It remained there for months, as I kept waiting for something to celebrate. Finally, someone stole it. I got the point. I had waited too long.

Dear God,
I give You
praise and thanks
for the blessings in my life.
May they not be diminished
by my lack of appreciation.
Teach me how to receive my good,
and support others in claiming theirs.
Amen

FOR MANY PEOPLE REACHING MIDLIFE, the role of parenting takes center stage. Raising children is an advanced spiritual practice, and that does not mean it's always easy. Holding children close when you're all the world to them is sometimes emotionally overwhelming; letting them go when they're ready to move away from you is overwhelming as well. And keeping the lines of communication open is often much easier said than done.

It's very different than it was when they were just cute little kids in their cute little outfits playing on cute little playdates. I see people with adorable babies, blissfully unaware that the day will come when they're so not in control, and I think, *Oh, honey, you wait.* But I say nothing. I just smile. Let them enjoy this while it lasts. Sooner than they think, they'll lose the unconditional adoration to which they've become accustomed.

Whatever you think you might be getting away with as a parent, trust me, you're not. Every mother and father meets the moment when a look in their child's eyes says, "Now I get it. I've figured you out." It's part of the individuation process that prepares the child to take the reins of their own lives: seeing the parent through the eyes of one who is no longer a child. Hopefully they'll stand on our shoulders where we got it right, breaking the cord where we got it wrong. We learn to respect the unfolding life of the son or daughter whose ultimate destiny is his or hers alone. A fiery life force moves from us into our children at a certain point; we can't hold on to the fire that used to be ours when it no longer is. Most of us watch with mixed emotions to see it ignite within them.

Watching our children grow up, like birds who really do fly away, is a profound rite of passage for both them and us. They become free in ways that only the young can be free. But we become free, too, in a way only someone who has raised their children to a certain age and watched them grow up can be. The child and the parent have both earned new wings.

We all have to follow the trajectory of our own soul growth. On one hand, I couldn't imagine how I'd feel no longer looking at the clock at 3:15 in the afternoon and thinking excitedly, "Oh, she'll be home soon!" (There's a fantastic way teenagers slam the door behind them when they come home from school, bellowing "I'm home!" with such confidence that it's the biggest news anybody's going to hear all day.) On the other hand, I know there will be new experiences in the future when we're no longer based in the same city, different from the ones we have now but hopefully just as wonderful.

Only when you allow someone else to grow do you get to grow too. And sometimes, of course, that means they grow away from you. Counterintuitively, the more you allow people to take the distance they need, the closer your bond often becomes with them.

I will never forget when my little girl was so tiny that I propped her up between pillows on my bed as I sat next to her and wrote. I think of that often when she's lying across the same bed now, chattering on after school about homework and history and life. These are the good old days, and believe me, I know it. Watching her one day, I began tearing up at the thought that she's growing up so fast; we won't be having these daily mother-daughter-plop-down-and-discuss-everything sessions after school each day for that much longer. But then my momentary sadness was interrupted by a vision just as beautiful as what was in front of me. I saw us plopped down right here again, but this time with another baby, as a new mother comes over to visit Grandma. The baby is gorgeous, the mother is ecstatic, and the grandma's pretty cool herself. Or so I saw in my mind's eye, and so I prayed.

Dear God,
Please take care of my precious child
as her path now leads her away from me.
May angels surround her
and may she find her way.
May my love for her
be a light that surrounds her
for all her living days.
Amen

Chapter Six

I Will Survive

A while back singer/songwriter Rupert Holmes had a hit song about a married couple who both took out personal ads, trying to find someone who wanted more adventure than was offered in their marriage. What they didn't know, of course—and found out when they answered each other's ad!—was that both of them wanted to do more exciting things than they were in the habit of doing together.

Years ago, I knew a man whose wife died, after which all he could do was just sit there crying, "I never took her on the trips she wanted to take. I didn't tell her often enough how much I loved her. There are so many things I should have done with her and didn't. . . ." It was tragic to see his eyes so open at a time when it was too late.

Many people, for whatever reasons, resist the grand adventure that love can be. It's one of those brass rings that is often right in front of us yet we don't grab on. It's one thing when we just don't feel the chemistry, when it's simply not the right person. But sometimes it *is* the right person—there *is* the energy—but we don't give the relationship the time, space, or attention it takes to cultivate what's good and see if it might turn into something great.

Once you're at a certain age, the idea of wasting any opportunity—particularly the opportunity to love—is seen as the self-inflicted wound that it is. You might as well just spit at God as turn away from the chance to really love. That's why love burns brightly at midlife; you're no longer under the delusion that the sparks which are flying here fly along every day. You tend to be more grateful, and more careful. Having been immature about love in the past, perhaps, you don't want to be immature about it now. Love is very serious business.

A friend of mine said to me once, "I used to be so afraid of committing to a woman for the rest of my life . . . but 'the rest of my life' doesn't sound like so long anymore!"

Many of us have wounds that now keep us from loving fearlessly. And our fears are understandable. Letting go your barriers to love that have accumulated over many years, in order to experience the love standing in front of you right now—such is the challenge of love at midlife. Here there are the most landmines, surely, and here can be the greatest joy.

Dear God,
Please melt
the walls in front of my heart.
Remove my fear
and restore my joy,
that I might love again.

Amen

ONE OF OUR BIGGEST FEARS, OBVIOUSLY, is the fear of abandonment. Clearly, it hits a primal wound when someone whose love has meant so much to us then changes his or her mind.

Metaphysically, what happens when we separate from a lover is that we reexperience our original separation from God—or at least the illusion that we could ever *be* separate. In fact, such a separation would be so shattering to the entire universe that the universe could no longer exist were it to be true. The truth is that our oneness with God, and with each other, is a fundamental, unalterable aspect of reality.

Not consciously realizing any of this, we displace our hunger for conscious contact with God onto our search for a romantic partner. Connection with a lover is intoxicating because it reminds us of our union with God; separation is so devastating because it triggers what it would feel like to be separate from Him. A terrible catch-22 develops: Feeling separate from God, I'm more hungry for you. But also, feeling separate from Him,

I'm not in my whole state. Being not in a whole state, I'm fractured—and thus more likely to *blow* it with you.

Love is a spiritual challenge, to be sure; sometimes a descent into hell and at its best a pure taste of heaven.

SOMETIMES IT'S THE ONE who takes away all our pain who then piles on even more of it.

I once had the most beautiful romance, or at least I thought so. Then one day it was simply gone. I had heard stories of people suddenly walking out on their families, never to return. But I always thought there must be more to it than that; surely it wasn't that simple. No one just got up one day and said, "It's over," and that was it. Or so I believed until it happened to me.

I'm one of those people who needs to *talk* . . . to process, to understand, to give and receive forgiveness if nothing else. But some people find all that talking at the end too much to take. Or perhaps the talking might expose too much. For whatever reason, it seems better for them to surgically remove the other person from their life, burn the bridge behind them, throw a bomb into a beautiful garden that could have been a friendship that lasted a lifetime.

This man had given me a gift. With him, I'd had the experience of a love that didn't conflict with my larger sense of mission for my life. For once there seemed to be no competition, no split, between my romantic life and my career. I didn't feel I was neglecting one in order to best serve the other, and for me that was new. Instead, I felt his love like a raft beneath me, on which I could just lie back serenely. Often before, I had felt as though the different elements of my life were like plates clanging against each other in a too-crowded dishwasher. Yet while he was there, there was no clanging. Things that usually seemed difficult weren't so hard to hold together. He'd meet what for me were the most stress-producing challenges with some line like, "Yeah, well, so what should we have for dinner?" and I would melt.

But then it ended, in an abrupt and unkind way. I, of course, had a choice to make. In the words of *A Course in Miracles,* I could be hostage to my ego or host to God. I knew that there is no letting go of others—the kind of release that frees not only them but you as well—without giving them your genuine blessing. It wouldn't be enough to just say, "I release you." I had to be able to say, "I release you and pray that you walk with angels. I release you and hope your dreams come true. I release you and wish you happiness." I resisted, as I was filled with resentment. But I prayed.

Soon after, I was reading *A Course in Miracles* and came across a truth that I needed to hear. I was reminded that all of us are equally holy in God's eyes . . . that whatever grievance I hold against another person has more to do with my own need to find blame than with anything they have done . . . and that regardless of what mistakes have been made by anyone in the past, in the present I can choose to see their innocence. Reading such things had the miraculous power to alchemize my emotions, to remove the painful impurities that, after all, weren't ruining *his* day—just mine!

The ego feasts on all this pain, like a scavenger dog delivering endless evidence of other people's cruelty, wrongdoing, injustices, and so forth. It's so tempting to monitor someone else's issues, leaving out of the equation that we ourselves might need to learn a few things. One of the most important gifts of any relationship is the gift of self-awareness. In *A Course in Miracles*, it says that "only what you are not giving can be lacking in any situation." Every relationship is a lesson learned. And in the final analysis, that is the reason for love: that one day we will *become* love. Everything that happens has a way of showing us how we're doing so far.

One morning I woke up thinking about him. I found myself saying a spontaneous prayer, no longer that God help me through this experience but that God help him. I'd known intellectually, of course, that this man's behavior at the end of our relationship was not that of a cruel person so much as that of a wounded one. But the intensity of my own pain had made me unable to see beyond the wound he'd inflicted on me to feel true compassion for his. And that was my lesson, clearly: to feel deeper compassion for someone else's wounds so I could then be healed of my own. Finally, on that particular morning, I could. I could imagine how much pain he would have had to be in, on some deep level, to so casually throw away the kind of connection we'd had. I thought of Gandhi's words: "Whenever you meet anyone, remember they are going through a great war." I could see that about him. I prayed for him, and despite my mixed feelings I wished him healed.

I could then see what perhaps had been the agreement forged between our souls. Like so many women, an anger at men—from unavailable fathers to unavailable lovers—had left a toughness in my heart that did not serve me well. Forgiving this man, praying for him, really wanting in my heart for him to be happy, I felt a shift inside myself. He stood for every man who had ever made me feel dismissed. Forgiving him helped me forgive them all. And then, in a deeper way, I was free.

The blessing was simply that I'd had the experience, and an experience cannot be possessed. It's there when it's there and it's gone when it's gone. Ultimately you come to realize that everything is yours and nothing is yours. As Helena says about her beloved Demetrius in Shakespeare's *A Midsummer Night's Dream:* "And I have found Demetrius like a jewel, / Mine own, and not mine own."

When you're young, you hold on tightly to love in the hopes that it will last forever. When you're older, you know you don't need to hold on because it *does* last forever. People come and they sometimes go. But love remains if it remains in you.

People often say, "I've been hurt so bad. How can I ever trust again?" But faith in love doesn't mean faith in someone's personality; it means faith in the changeless nature of love itself, which is in fact the Love of God. Faith in love isn't just faith in another person; ultimately, it's faith in ourselves as well. It's faith in our capacity to discern and our capacity to forgive. It means faith in our capacity to love fiercely, yet with the full understanding that all form is temporary even at its best.

True love is always a risk, in that sense. But the universe isn't invested in giving us what we want. It's invested in teaching us how to love. And if we bless others when they're with us, but withhold our blessing if and when they leave, then we have not yet learned how to love. A blessing that isn't constant is not a blessing.

What we trust is the will of God. We're brought into each other's lives on divine assignment, spirit working through the subconscious mind to draw us to people with whom we have the greatest opportunity for soul growth. But that doesn't mean that the lessons will always be easy. In fact, someone might have been brought into our lives so we can master the lesson of discernment—in other words, to teach us what to turn *away* from.

Sometimes it's an experience of what you do not ultimately want that teaches you what you *do* want. Sometimes it's the one who shatters you who releases you to your greatest capacity for love. Something didn't turn out to be what you hoped for, but perhaps that was the point. It was a relationship that released you to you, thus setting you on a higher path. True love can't come until you know yourself, and you couldn't know yourself until certain appetites were blasted out of you.

You might have had an appetite for the less than committed because you weren't ready to *be* committed. Now, having been run from, you are ready to stop running. Now, having been stung, you are ready to stop stinging. And now a true love—someone who neither stings nor runs nor is attracted to pain—is on their way to meet you. In the words or the Persian poet Rumi, "Out of a shattered open heart springs a fountain of fiery sacred passion that will never run dry."

Don't skip a beat. Perfume your skin. Make ready your house. Prepare your heart.

Perhaps you were let down by a love of this world, so you would learn at last to lean only on God.

Dear God,
I surrender to You
my past relationships.
Teach me how to forgive,
dear God,
that I might be weighed down no longer.
I release the ones who have wounded me:
May they now find their joy.
May I be forgiven
for the wounds I've inflicted.
May all of us find true peace.
Amen

THE PROBLEM WITH *NOT* LEANING ON GOD is that we then tend to lean inordinately on other people. Failing to embrace a love that will always be there for us, we become vulnerable to ones that won't be.

I remember a television show that was very popular when I was a little girl called *Father Knows Best.* Every time the teenage daughter walked into a room, her father gave her a huge smile and exclaimed, "Why hello, Princess!" Being so deeply adored by her father at that age, a girl's brain would be imprinted with an emotional propensity for men who treat her in a similarly adoring way. Healthy male attention would feel natural to her; she'd grow up knowing what it looks like and how she should respond to it.

But if male attention is missing, then the girl grows up in many cases to be a woman who either deflects such a comment because it's so alien to her, or goes in the opposite direction and practically turns it into a marriage proposal! Either way, there's a void where a genuine sense of her female self should be. And boy, is an inauthentic person a sucker for an inauthentic person.

A woman like that would be particularly vulnerable to emotional charlatans—the "charmers" who say exactly the right thing and know a fair amount of poetry, but from whom there's rarely a responsible follow-through to their protestations of devotion. He too was almost always a wounded child. Something made it necessary for him, when young, to learn performance as a survival skill. For whatever reason, he came to feel at a tragically early age that deceit rather than authenticity was a normal mode of being. Conscious connection to his own deeper truth was superseded by a need to find whatever words or behavior would help him survive a traumatic moment. Life taught him to behave falsely—not how to present himself as he truly is, in touch with his honest feelings and deeper truth—but rather to display with lightning speed whatever behavior gives him a short-term emotional advantage.

Someone who learned the subtleties of human manipulation at an early age tends to be very good at it by the time he's an adult. Such a person simply lacks integrity; not because he's a bad human being, but because he was knocked out of his spiritual center as a child and hasn't yet learned to reclaim it. As a child, he was a victim; as an adult, however, he'll be held accountable for his behavior one way or another. As a friend once said to me, "The universe keeps a perfect set of books."

How many times have we excused someone's unacceptable behavior with lines like, "But inside, he's just a wounded little boy"? To which a girlfriend of mine once responded, "So was Hitler." The fact that I have compassion for you doesn't mean I shouldn't delete you from my phone.

Damaged people damage people. They're also attracted to other damaged people. So we should all beware.

Those such as the man and woman described above would easily be drawn to each other, as their neuroses form a perfect fit. He's a performer extraordinaire, and she's easily taken in by a great performance. Their egos' intention is that they trigger each other's wounds, but God's intention is that they *heal* each other's wounds. Which it will be is up to both of them. Whoever is willing to do the work in a relationship, seeing it as their own opportunity for self-healing, will receive the blessing whether the other person makes that choice or not. And ultimately, all of us will get there; lessons we haven't learned will just keep coming around until we do.

Healing can hurt—whether it's the healing of having to face the shame of humiliation, or the pain of having to turn our backs on someone whose patterns are unhealthy for us to be around though we love them still. Either way, the pain of the healing is far preferable to the pain of remaining at the effect of a neurotic pattern.

The woman will find, if she searches, that while her worldly daddy wasn't always there, her Heavenly Father is there for her always; never fails to adore her; and has created her whole, which she will always be. The man will discover—if he continues his spiritual quest—that the patterns of deceit that he learned so early and have now become forces over which he seems to have no control, can and will be healed as he acknowledges them, owns them, and prays that they be lifted.

Will the man and woman above get past their wounds? Will she grow strong enough in her sense of true self to lose all attraction to false romantics, preferring authentic love before the ersatz version? Will he at last feel bad enough about the hurt he causes others to ask for God's help in changing his behavior? Both must choose. The one who learns and grows will mature and ripen with age. The one who doesn't will just grow old.

Dear God,
Please heal my romantic wounds
that I might give and receive true love.
Teach me how to let love in
and how to let it stay.
Amen

In actress Ellen Burstyn's superb memoir, *Lessons in Becoming Myself,* she describes how, after a dramatic, decades-long string of husbands and lovers, she found herself taking a 25-year break—repeat: 25 *years*—before ultimately finding the healthy, wholesome romance she'd always wanted. She didn't even date during her romantic hiatus, so sure was she that any liaison she developed would just be a reflection of the same painful patterns she'd played out in her relationships until then.

Let's call this a "sex-and-love fast." Few people think of it that way when they're going through it, of course. While we're experiencing it, we just feel it's a "dry spell" or even the "end of all that"; we might think it's happening because we're older now, so we don't attract lovers as easily anymore. But the truth is often that we declared a halt to romance on a subconscious level, regardless of how much the conscious mind protests that "I'd love to meet someone."

Why? As a middle-aged friend of mine once responded when I asked her if she was seeing anyone, "No. I can't stand who I become when I'm in a relationship. I'd rather not even do it." Once you see that in every relationship you've encountered the same demon—your *own*—you realize that until you deal with that demon, you'll never find true love. For the demon blocks it. This demon takes various forms in your arsenal of self-sabotage: insecurity, lack of boundaries, jealousy, dishonesty, anger, control, neediness, or whatever other form of personal inauthenticity leads you time and time again to either attract the bad ones or blow it with the good ones. It is naïve to underestimate that demon's power.

After one of her romances went desperately sour, a friend once told me, "Another one like that would kill me." I understood what she meant, and so can most people. There comes a time when you feel like the high of romance isn't worth the pain of its demise; when the risk of a romantic disaster outweighs the thrill of the ride. And that time is . . . you guessed it . . . more often than not around midlife.

Why? Because you've been through enough to know what can go wrong. You might have experienced enough disasters to be desperate not to repeat another. And that's the challenge: You know enough to be wise now, but you also know enough to be scared. Discernment and clarity aren't just luxuries anymore; they're required if you're to find your right path and keep your peace of mind. And a definite win in the clarity department is that your body isn't screaming for it all the time the way it once did. Your body isn't so upset at the thought that you're taking a break; it might even welcome the chance for some downtime. There's a wildness to young love that had its place, as well as its heartbreaks and joys. The search for love at midlife is still wild, but it's wildness of a different sort.

The yearning for love remains, but it alchemizes into something less personal. Not less personal in the sense that you don't want an intimate conversation or a warm body holding you close, just less personal in the sense that life has forced you to see beyond the illusion that any human being can erase all your pain. You realize the romantic mythology we were all brought up with is like a computer file that has been corrupted. Until that file has been removed and then replaced by another, no matter what we do, our ultimate outcome will be tainted.

This doesn't mean you don't still crave love—the craving itself never stops. As a matter of fact, at just the point when we've had enough, the very fact that we *have* had enough is what causes our breakthrough into the awareness that sets us free. As it's said in Alcoholics Anonymous, "Every problem comes bearing its own solution." It's often when love has hurt the most, that we're forced to look at how and why we set ourselves up for all that pain.

So you go on a fast. All of a sudden, your phone stops ringing. Like Ellen Burstyn, you're forced to cleanse your palate.

Burstyn came to understand that her negative relationship patterns were reflections of her childhood wounds, which she'd have to reenact until she healed them. So do we all. Until that work is done on some level, there is no getting off the wheel of suffering. Our subconscious minds aren't wrong in cutting us off from love and sex for a while, as the inner work is being done and deeply absorbed into our system. The fast isn't something we do to isolate; it's something we do to survive.

First there was childhood, and the wounding that occurred then. Then there was young adulthood, and the disasters that occurred because of our childhood wounds. And then there's midlife, when it's time to deal at last with what happened in childhood *and* in young adulthood. Midlife is the time to heal, so our hearts can finally be delivered from the past and released to the fullness of what love can be right now.

When you see a lot of middle-aged individuals at personal-growth seminars, it's not because they're done with love and this is their only entertainment now. Often, they have memories that might shock the younger people around them. Whenever you see an older person, you might want to subtract 40 years, and imagine who they were then. Midlife is not a time to simply dwell on our memories of love and the demons we encountered there; it's time to develop the skill at last to send our demons back to hell.

Sometimes you wonder if you missed your window. Ellen Burstyn writes that she remembered feeling, *Now that I know I am ready at last to love well, I fear it is too late.* With that sentiment, she echoes the fears of many. Yet that's just a typical, last-ditch effort of the demon to deter us, a common pain that often pops up in our head in that one minute before the miracle.

Once your mind and heart are realigned—when the broken self you became in childhood is no longer manifesting broken relationships—then you're ready at last to love again. Compassion, integrity, truthfulness, generosity, and graciousness become key elements in your new romantic skill set. You come to see what you did wrong in the past and to forgive yourself, to understand other people's actions and, where needed, forgive them too. You are humbled at last into your purity and grace.

In the Epilogue of her book, Burstyn describes how she finally met the man of her dreams, and I finished the last page thinking, *Now I want to read the sequel!* I'd read hundreds of pages about the horrors of her past; now I wanted to know what finally getting it right would look and feel like to her.

Just as certain foods need to marinate, our romantic skills need years sometimes to come together in all their richness. I asked Burstyn what it's like now, to finally feel that she loves and is loved well. "What's different?" I asked her.

"For starters," she said, "there is much more respect and much less judgment. Conversations don't escalate into arguments, and arguments don't escalate into violence." She paused. "And now I know how to let a man be."

In our younger years, we often had love, but we didn't know what to do with it. Then sometimes, after what can be a very long time in the romantic wilderness, we find love again or love finds us. And this time, we *do* know what to do. That wilderness—that fast—was not the end of anything. It was our romantic salvation.

Dear God,
Please reveal to me
the glory of those you send for me to love.
Help me be still within myself
So I can let them come to me.
Help me to not abandon myself
So I will not abandon them.
Amen

I ALWAYS HATE IT WHEN I'M ASKED TO FILL out an official form of some kind that includes the options "single," "married," or "divorced." I always leave that section blank, as my way of saying, "That's none of your damn business."

I think I feel that way because it seems too personal. It feels like an emotional identity theft, giving someone permission to make assumptions about me based on such external categories. (Calm down, Marianne. This is a *dental* form.)

Which is not to say, of course, that whether we're married or single doesn't matter. It's just to say that the deeper issues of love are not about form but content. The problem I see most often blocking the romantic impulse is a stifled sense of self: Many men aren't really sure how to be men, and many women aren't really sure how to be women. Our generational detour into an ambisexual wasteland was part of what emotionally stunted many of us for years. When a woman thinks that she can overdo her "masculine self" and a man will still want her, or a man thinks that he can overdo his "feminine self" and a woman will still want him, then all manner of confusion leads to all manner of pain. That delusional trend has begun to self-correct, but the collective wound is not yet fully healed. It's one of those many areas where our parents sometimes had it right—for the wrong reasons, perhaps, but in ways we didn't realize, they had it right.

My mother was a broad. If she had an opinion, you knew it. If she didn't like something, she'd let you hear about it. And my father never seemed to think that he had the right to stop her from expressing herself. He never seemed to want to. *However* . . . there was a limit that he sometimes set, not to her self-expression but to any discomfort it might be causing him.

My father never called my mother by her name, ever. He always called her "Sweetheart." But every once in a while—not frequently, but at those rare times when something she was going on about was stirring tension he was not okay with—my father simply looked at her and said simply, "Sophie Ann." And my mother stopped. That was it. She grew silent. It took me years and tears to understand what a lucky woman my mother was. He loved her for who and what she was, *and* he had boundaries.

For a woman to be strong and wild and creatively rambunctious, she can't afford to be with a partner who stifles her, invalidates her, or punishes her for being who she is. That being said, a woman is blessed by the presence of someone who can say, in a way that doesn't withhold his affection or undermine her confidence, "Are you sure you want to go that far?"

For many women, our deepest craving is for a place to relax. The mistake we make is when we're looking for that in a lover instead of first finding it within ourselves. When we do look within, embracing our Divine Partner instead of prowling the world for an earthly one, our very state of being magnetizes love. The tricks of the ego are cunning and cruel: We're looking for someone to make us feel okay, when as soon as we know we just *are* okay, then the lover arrives at our door.

Nothing is more powerful than accepting what *is*, including ourselves. Too often we inquire how we can change a situation, when we should be asking how we can dwell within it in the highest possible way. Who knew that personal impeccability has its own kind of sex appeal.

If you're single and would like a partner, you'll only attract one when you've mastered the lessons of singleness. Don't ask how you can "get" a lover. Ask how you can be the coolest person in the world—and when that happens, you'll enjoy the experience so much it won't even matter whether the perfect someone notices you or not. Which means, of course, that they will.

I did a lot of research so that I could report back on that.

One of the most insidiously self-sabotaging questions is, "Why can't I meet the right person?" It implies that there is someone out there, maybe in Mongolia or someplace, and if only you knew where he or she was, then you could pop over on the next flight.

But since metaphysically nothing is outside of us—everything we experience is a reflection of what's going on in our head—there's no point in flying to Mongolia if we're not yet ready to show up for our ideal partner in the highest possible way. And once we *are* ready, we needn't go anywhere because he or she will simply appear. Once we've grieved what we have to grieve, looked at what we have to look at, and then finally come home to ourselves, he or she will be there.

Whenever people have stood up in my lectures—and it has been often—to say their heartbreak is that they haven't yet found a mate, I usually find myself saying,

"Tell me the truth; I know you know it. What do you do that keeps love at bay?"

Often the room gasps, as though I've said something confrontational. And perhaps I have: I've asked a person to confront him- or herself. I've suggested that they take full responsibility for their own experience. And more often than not, after a pause, I'm met with an honest and illuminating answer:

"I act needy."

"I attract men, but then I start acting like a man myself, so they leave. I'm not very feminine."

"I get jealous."

"I get angry."

"I'm controlling."

"I'm so desperate to have kids and men can feel it."

Then I usually say something like this: "Ah. Well, then isn't it wonderful that your great love isn't here yet? You can handle this now, so you don't ruin another good opportunity!"

So it's not only understandable why those people are single—it's *good* that they are! This is their time to get ready. Time to do the work, internally and externally, that goes along with preparing yourself as the gift you really are—not as an assorted set of fragmented emotions, unhealed neuroses, and broken dreams from an unforgiven past.

The most important thing to work on, always, is the nature of our thoughts. Whenever we believe that a situation is lacking, we create more lack. Why? Because lack is our core belief. *Believing* you lack, you *attract* more lack. *I lack love in my life* is not a thought that invites a partner. *What I've got is hot* goes further.

And one thing we should never do is believe statistics. Years ago, I saw a major news magazine article that said woman over a certain age had a better chance of being killed by a terrorist than finding love at midlife. But guess what? That magazine ended up taking back its pronouncement! We *do* have a chance! *Oh, thank you!* So we learned something important from that little turnaround: We need to watch what we read. Be aware of what junk you let into your consciousness. And don't expect the voices of the world to know one damn thing about what's happening in your universe.

A girlfriend of mine once remarked, "I hate being single because when I walk into a party alone, I feel like everyone thinks I'm pathetic and is feeling sorry for me." I told her that this was just her thought and nothing else. "For all you know," I said, "they assume you're meeting some rock star after the party." Midlife is the time to stop giving one moment's thought to other people's opinions anyway. Let them think whatever they want to think. It's *your* thoughts that create your experience.

Love is attracted to the master at love. It does not ask, "What's your age?" Nor does it ask, "How long did it take you to learn all this?" It only asks whether you're ready. And when you are, then it will come.

It can take a lot of years before you arrive at love's door with little or no baggage. There might have been struggles galore making all the shifts, from neediness to self-confidence, controlling to surrendered, anxious to lighthearted, demanding to grateful, overreactive to nonreactive, critical to supportive, blaming to forgiving, chaotic to calm. But once you arrive, you *really* arrive.

Someone once said to me, "You're everything I've ever wanted." I turned my face and uttered under my breath, "Honey, if ya only knew . . . !"

ONCE YOU'VE LOVED, you do stand a chance of having encountered the demons that surround it: someone's fear, someone's lies, someone's betrayal. You can go forward now in timidity and fear, with an energy that reads, "I come with *lots* of baggage." Or you can go forward with the energy that only the experience of love in all its vicissitudes can give, an energy that reads, "I have seen some demons, but I stared them down." No one gets excited about some bitter woman they met last night. But there's a powerful magnetism to those who have chosen *not* to be bitter. Bitterness is a repellant. it's a surefire way to keep love at bay.

And there's nothing to be bitter about once you take responsibility for your own mistakes. Among other things, experience teaches you how to make better choices. If unworthy opportunities are offered you, you'll know to give them a pass. Your hard-earned wisdom makes you more likely to say no to untrustworthy offers, and a wise but openhearted yes to good ones. No book or school could have taught you that.

Sometimes it's the pain of love that transforms you into someone who has the courage to take it on. You come to thank God for the lessons you learned, no matter how they came to you or what they felt like at the time. So *what* if you're not young anymore; you have so much more skill now, and so much less fear. Now at last you are ready for love. Bring it on.

Chapter Seven

In the Midnight Hour

I remember the moment the doctor told me. I was standing in my kitchen, not having bothered to emotionally prepare myself for the call. I'd had light menstrual periods for years, and I realized the chances were good that, although I was still quite young, the end might have already come.

And it had. The doctor had gotten back my numbers. He put it bluntly: "You're done."

The room spun around me; I felt too weak to stand. I sat down slowly and the tears began. After all the years you work so hard to keep from getting pregnant, you suddenly find that you couldn't get pregnant anymore if you tried. In that moment you regret every damned act of birth control you'd engaged in your entire life. Something miraculous occurs in your body every month, and then it's gone. It is simply gone.

Even if they never wanted children, I've known few menopausal women who escaped the sorrow, deep and ancient, of realizing they were done. We didn't realize how much it meant to us that we *could* produce children, until we realized we could not. I remember a poster that was popular years ago, with a cartoon character of a woman exclaiming, "Oh my gosh, I forgot to have children!" Many of us took so long to grow up that we were nearing middle age before we even took the subject seriously.

One day I attended a luncheon where I was sitting next to a man about my age, who was delightedly telling stories about his teenaged stepdaughters. He commented that he had never had children of his own and felt so blessed to be a stepparent now.

Sensing his joy and absolute wonder at what the girls had brought into his life, I looked at him for a moment and simply said, "We were so damned stupid." He looked back at me, clearly understanding what I meant, and nodded slowly. He would have wanted children. I would have wanted four.

That says it: *We were so damned stupid.*

Someone once asked me what greatness I thought my daughter was destined to achieve, and I responded, "First of all, I think she'll have a big happy family." They thought I was joking. I was not.

I watched with awe when the baton of voluptuousness passed to my 17-year-old daughter. Of course I didn't want to mimic a 17-year-old's attractiveness, but I did want to hold on to my own as best I could. There's a certain psycho-erotic quality that a woman never wants to lose;

the feeling that any night could be a magic night and you want to be ready for it if this one is.

I remember the hormones of youth. I remember when every cell of my body screamed, "Get a man! Get *any* man!" Later they were just as apt to say, "Whatever. I don't care." My body stopped being a slave to itself the way it once was, but my soul took things to a whole new place.

It's natural that there are years when the thought of sex is pretty much everyone's preoccupation; the species can't propagate unless young people move the process forward. But sometimes it's when the urge for sex becomes a little less urgent that the urge for love becomes more pure. The urge for connection itself is ageless; what changes is our understanding of what connection *means*. Sometimes people know a lot about sex but not much at all about love.

In the realm of the body, something starts to cool off as we age. But in the realm of the spirit, age is when things are just heating up. Mature women are pursued not just for their bodies but for their *knowing*. A man recognizes, however unconsciously, that a woman's love is an initiation into his own manhood. On a physical level, that initiation can mean something as crude as a ride in the backseat of a car. But on a spiritual level, it's the result of an internal connection that sex itself can't guarantee. For this, a man needs more than a woman. He needs a priestess. Every woman has an inner priestess, but she often takes a few decades to emerge. A priestess is fierce—particularly in bed.

If what you're up to is producing babies, then obviously the younger woman has the goods. With a younger woman, a man can conceive a child. But with a priestess, he is often more likely to conceive the man he wants to be. Physically, a man spreads his seed; spiritually, a woman spreads hers. Ultimately, we impregnate each other and then we are both reborn. (The same is true with same sex relationships, of course.) When a man has spent magic time with a woman mature and wise enough to have entered her priestess years, he's the one who becomes pregnant with something. The new breed of priestesses have miraculous powers, calling forth a new breed of man.

ONE DAY MY DAUGHTER came home and told me I just had to hear this great new song. It was a cover of Bob Dylan's "Lay, Lady, Lay." I explained to her that in my day, we listened to the *real* "Lay, Lady, Lay." And in my case, as I'm sure is true for thousands of others as well, we did a whole lot more than just listen. I've asked myself often in the last few years, "What did my mother think we were *doing* on those afternoons?"

I read a quote once that no matter how old we are, the music we most relate to is the music of our youth. In my case, that's definitely true. And the songs I remember most are the songs I fell in love to. From Joan Armatrading to Jefferson Airplane to Van Morrison, there are phrases of songs that remind me of things, beautiful things, that were some of the sweetest moments of my life.

And why were they so sweet? Because, along with the birth of my daughter, they took me to a place where there was no separation between myself and someone else.

And that was real. The love affairs we had in our youth were not unreal, so much as the personality structures we went on to develop afterward were not containers for that much reality. Some of what we call "mature" in our society is spiritually regressive.

I WAS SITTING NEXT TO A MAN on an airplane once, who told me that he and his wife were excited about a new business venture. For the first time in their marriage, they were going to be working together. They had refurbished a carriage house in back of their home and had turned it into an office. All of this seemed to them like a fabulous next step in both their careers and their relationship.

As he told me of their plans, I think he saw me choke on my red wine.

"What?" he asked.

"Nothing," I responded, aware that I didn't even know this man, and had no business giving him unsolicited advice. But he persisted. He asked. And once you do that with me, expect opinions.

"Well, what I've learned," I told him, "is that when a woman is working, she's in a masculine mode. But that same mode that works so well at work needs to transition to a feminine mode if she wants to be as successful at love as she is at work." Again, I've researched this.

"Go on . . . ," he said.

"So it probably seems great to you now, that you and your wife will be able to just walk the little path from your office to your kitchen and keep the same conversation going while you're preparing dinner that you were having at the office."

"Is that bad?" he asked.

"No, it's not bad," I said, "except possibly for your marriage. You've taken the psychic gestalt of a business partnership and literally given it the run of your house. And in time, that will include your bedroom."

"Whoa," he said. Men get very alert when the subject turns to sex. "So I shouldn't work with my wife?"

"I didn't say that!" I responded. "That's not for me to say. But I do know this: If this kind of thinking makes sense to you—if you feel that you and your wife want to protect the erotic quality of your marriage from encroachment by a business mentality—then I would suggest you take 30 minutes apart from each other between office hours and evening hours. She needs at least that much time to switch psychically into another mode. Meditation, walking, soft music, candles, bubble baths, whatever her soul craves as a balm to her nervous system—that time should be ritualistically built into your lifestyle, or you're going to start finding that a businesswoman has shown up in your bed where an erotic goddess used to be."

Weeks later I received a thank-you note from him. And after that, one from his wife . . . !

Romantic love is a force of nature. Like an ancient goddess, it likes to receive gifts. It must be honored, respected, protected, and cherished. Otherwise, it simply leaves.

Dear God,
Please make me
a master at love.
Reveal to me its mysteries
and give to me its magic.
May I enchant and be enchanted,
but never ensnare or be ensnared.
Show me the holiness of love.
Amen

A FRIEND TOLD ME HER DAUGHTER was getting married at the age of 40.

"That's great!" I said. "Is she madly in love?"

"Well, I don't know if it's *like* that at forty," she responded.

I thought to myself, *Wow, why not?* What, like 40 is *old* or something?

The age of our cells has nothing to do with our ability to magnetize or hold on to love. Midlife is not the time to say, "Oh well, I'll just settle for something comfortable now," and simplistically conclude that the years of heat are behind us. That heat was not a function of our age. It might move around from chakra to chakra, but heat will always be heat.

Love doesn't lose its edge and become boring as you get older unless *you* do. If anything, age makes you more able to appreciate things in others that you used to be unable to see because you were so busy looking at yourself. Until you inhabit the entirety of your being, you keep seeking your completion in someone else. And that will never work, of course. Romance isn't here to complete your universe but to expand it. That's why seeking a more expanded space of spiritual understanding, completely separate from any search for romantic love, actually prepares you for it. Love finds you more easily, and you're less likely to be thrown off your center when it does. Being grounded in God's love, you're less afraid of human love. Closeness to God is alignment with our true self, and alignment with our true self makes us more comfortable within the earthiness of human intimacy.

Accumulated experience of the world both breaks your heart and opens it. I remember lying in the dark one night right after a school shooting, when my grief for the victims' families felt like more than I could bear. I turned to my love and, for just one moment, felt an exquisite understanding of the profound juxtaposition of pain and pleasure that lies at the heart of the human experience. I loved in a different way before I understood suffering. Age wears you down, but as it does, it softens you as well. I knew in that moment that there are no guarantees. There is no certain bulwark against human suffering. Neither this relationship, nor any other circumstance, could possibly protect me against the potential for heartbreak; whatever valleys are my fate will occur no matter what. But there is, when we are open to the experience, the glorious beauty of an appreciated now. When we no longer take the good in life for granted, we have a humility and gratitude that more than compensate for what no longer remains of our innocence. Innocence leaves, but love remains. There is nothing to do with this but receive its truth. I opened my arms and I drank him in.

MANY WOMEN IN MIDLIFE are confronted with the question, "But is he too young for me?"

Beyond obvious proprieties, I don't think it should matter how old your lover is any more than it should matter how old your doctor, teacher, or car-insurance salesperson is. What matters is the spiritual connection that brings our hearts together. Every relationship has a natural arc, a time that's perfect for the lessons that the relationship is here to teach us. *A Course in Miracles* says people are brought together for as long a period of time as serves their maximal soul growth. Some relationships are long and some are short. Love will never bow to time because love is real and time is not. A moment of true love is more important to some of us than decades of domestic time-share.

Love is an adventure of the soul, whether as a love affair that is short but intense, or as a marriage that lasts until death do us part. In the words of Ram Dass, we are brought into each other's lives "for a reason, a season, or a lifetime." It isn't the length of time, but rather the depth of knowing and forgiveness and growth that occurs, which determines the meaning of a connection between two people. I love the Joni Mitchell lyric that love is souls touching souls. Some people have slept together for 30 years but their souls have never touched. By some estimation, theirs is still a successful marriage . . . but there are many ways to estimate love.

I once knew a man who was younger than I was chronologically, but much more firmly grounded in the truth of his being than I was in mine. I kept up this inauthentic mantra about how he was much too young for me, until one day I realized that the quizzical look on his face wasn't disappointment, it was disrespect. He had expected more of me. He expected me to be more honest.

What a convenient front for my fear it was to go on and on about how he hadn't had his babies yet, and since I couldn't give him those, then of course I wasn't the woman for him. "For a lifetime, you're probably right," he said. "But I didn't ask you for a lifetime. I asked you for Saturday night."

But how can I relax on Saturday night, I thought, *when I already know that this is a limited run?* I saw an episode of *Sex and the City* where that's called "expiration dating": You know in advance that there's a date past which you can't continue this. It took a while for me to realize that that had never stopped me from enjoying yogurt, so it didn't have to stop me from enjoying love either!

So I gave the young man a chance—as though I had so much to teach him, you see. And the irony, which was no irony at all to him but simply an obvious point, was that he, carrying so much less fear than I, came to the experience with more wisdom and strength. Whatever I had in accumulated knowledge, he bested with his more open mind: fewer rules, fewer limits, fewer affectations of knowing things that can't be known. It wasn't I who was the guru at love here; it was he. I thought he might be blessed by the love of someone more knowing than he, but I think I was more blessed to be loved by someone more *unknowing* than I. People are matched perfectly for the gifts they bring to each other, and sometimes it's those who teach us when *not* to reason who are as important as those who teach us how to. Knowledge has many dimensions. *A Course in Miracles* states that love restores reason and not the other way around.

Sometimes the value of a liaison with a younger person is that they remind us of what's eternal, still buried within us by obscured by the passage of years. They bring energy like the sun breaking through, after too much fog and rain had made us think the light might not ever return. They bring the sun because they still *are* the sun. Having not yet experienced their own late afternoon, they don't trigger the grief you feel over what happened during yours.

A relationship might not be something that lasts a lifetime, but that doesn't mean it's not a temple experience. The sanctity of a connection is determined by the respect and honor with which we show up for it. People are drawn to people whom they can learn from, and intimacy is a deep learning. Years together can be a deep learning, and three days in Paris where all you do is eat and sleep and make love and pray and talk about everything that's ever happened to you can also be a deep learning. The only thing that ruins that one is when someone doesn't know how to let what happened in Paris be simply that. It takes a high level of spiritual as well as emotional evolution to be able to go deep with someone with whom the connection is best kept limited in time.

I'm not justifying casual sex here; the sex in this case would be anything but casual. This isn't that "What happens in Vegas stays in Vegas." It's that "What happened in Paris will stay in our hearts to bless us forever."

THERE ARE MANY MANSIONS in the romantic house of love. The exchange is uniquely wonderful with someone who knows the lyrics to the same songs you do. I think of one who walked the path with me when it was smooth and when it was rocky, when it was cool to know me and when it was cool to put me down, when I was laughing like a loon and when I was crying like a child. He is the one who has *seen* me. That is the ultimate value, I think, of relationships that move through the years without dissolving. Someone bears witness to your life. You don't experience yourself in a vacuum; someone else knows your story. They were as excited as you when something marvelous happened to you, and they never said, "I told you so," when you did something stupid you would later regret. They have faith in the longer narrative of your life. They've seen you grow from your losses as well as your wins.

The key to long-term relationships is letting someone be different today than they were yesterday. I think one of the main reasons for divorce is when couples don't create the emotional permission for each other to change. When people say, "We grew apart," it's often a sign that when they entered the marriage, their emotional contract didn't include this clause: "I'll let you change. You'll let me change." Sometimes the problem isn't that someone starts to grow in a new or different direction. It's that they don't invite their partner to participate, or the partner invalidates the change out of fear that it will take their spouse away. Sometimes things that pull people apart didn't have to.

At midlife, we're different people than we were when we were younger. Was it that someone "got married too young," or just that the partners in a relationship didn't know how to give each other permission to grow? People who don't change over time grow boring, and so do relationships. There's a huge change when a child becomes an adolescent, just as there's a huge change when adolescence ends. Why should we think there is less of a change as we enter midlife?

At midlife we all need to shed our skin and grow a new one. The soul hungers for a chance to expand itself. The tragedy between partners is when they don't know enough to honor this need, recognizing that it carries within it a chance to regreen a relationship.

I once knew a man who left his wife because he felt that he couldn't become *himself* in the marriage. He felt that he couldn't find his manhood within the context of their connection, as if she took up too much of the oxygen. He felt that in leaving her, he was going through a male initiation of sorts. Then and only then could he become the man he wanted to be.

But I felt in observing them that perhaps the truest initiation into his manhood would have been if, within the context of the marriage, he'd owned his own power enough to simply tell her to back off. A real man does set boundaries. A real man does demand his own psychic space. A real man does not let a woman dominate or control him. But a real man *claims* all that for himself; he doesn't just slink away and call leaving his marriage some assumption of male power.

Sometimes marriages are simply over—the maximum opportunity for learning has occurred, and it's time to let go—but sometimes people leave for no other reason than that their spouses aren't providing them with what only they can provide for themselves. The fact that a relationship is reminding you that you're not strong enough yet isn't of itself a *bad* thing. It's part of the value of the relationship that it's showing you to yourself. Moving on to another situation where you're stuck in the same pattern, but just pretend you're not, has never in my experience brought freedom from the pattern itself.

I've gained a lot in my life from moving on, when moving on was the call of my soul. I've gained just as much from staying in the struggle with self while standing still, when my soul made it clear that this was where I belonged for now . . . that the real problem was not with him but with me. And it is incredible, once you've made the breakthrough or made the change, when the person in front of you is the same one who was there before.

I once had a relationship with a man who told me often, "You're so hard to please." It was an ongoing issue that became a major one, as I'd always find a way to create a problem where there didn't have to be one. I got the point and sought to address within myself why I was behaving in such a self-defeating way. I asked for God's help, tried to snap out of it, and modified my behavior as best I could. One day many months later, I asked my friend for another serving of half-and-half in my coffee, to which he responded laughingly, "You're so hard to please." I had made it. I had changed. And he was still there.

Dear God,
I surrender to You my relationships.
Please purify my thoughts about them,
so only love remains.
In this, and in all things, dear God,
may Your Will alone
be done.
Show me the truth and innocence in others
That I might see it in myself.
Remove my blindness to the beauty in others,
And teach me how to love.
Amen

Chapter Eight

Abraham, Martin, and John

Dear God,
At this time of global peril,
may I be a conduit of Your miracles.
Heal me that I
might heal others,
and help bring forth
a more beautiful world.
Amen

During his second term in office, President Bill Clinton proposed a national conversation about race. People tried their best to live up to the proposition, but soon enough the idea seemed to fizzle. From a transformational perspective—one that recognizes the importance of psychological, emotional, and spiritual factors, as well as material ones—this came as no surprise. You can't have a real "conversation" about race—one that's authentic and meaningful, with any hope of real breakthrough—unless some of the people involved have a chance to express anger that's been built up over hundreds of years.

Having led spiritual support groups for more than 20 years, I've had a bit of experience facilitating the kind of sacred space that allows for deep conversation. A unique energy must be brought forth in such groups, ensuring the emotional safety and well-being of all its participants. Most of us have felt this kind of energy in therapy, during religious ritual, or what have you. It's a distinctly different vibration from normal conversation, stemming from a different set of brain waves.

When Mary was looking for her son Jesus, she found him in the temple. And there was a reason for that. No soul finds any soul except in sacred space.

Within that space, all is revealed—total communication is given and received, and miracles occur naturally. Until we reach that depth of dialogue within ourselves and with others, there can be no deeper breakthroughs regarding our most urgent problems. What will *not* solve today's problems is conventional thought. What will *not* solve today's problems is old tried-and-no-longer-true formulas. What will *not* solve today's problems is endless attack and defense. What will *not* solve today's problems is shallow conversation.

What *will* solve today's problems is new consciousness, from which will emerge new thinking and new hope. The planet needs a new story, and so do we.

Who would be better to help create a new story for the planet than those of us who just happen to be involved with creating a new story for ourselves? A problem of mid-life is the temptation to be redundant, simply imitating ourselves by doing the same things we've always done but with less verve. But the pulse of the moment—both personally and globally—is to let go now of what needs to be let go, to disenthrall ourselves of what used to be, and embrace a radically new kind of life. It is there for us. It's there for us as individuals, and it's there for us as a species. It's alive in our imagination, and we can claim it if we wish to. Each of us is coded to play a maximally effective role helping to change the world, to the extent to which we are willing to *be changed.*

I was once privy to a fascinating moment at a private party, where I saw the musical producer and performer Babyface sit strumming a guitar and singing his song "Change the World," while former mayor of Atlanta, UN ambassador, and civil-rights legend Andrew Young sat a few feet away, listening and staring out into the distance. One man sang of wanting to change the world, while the other had memories of how much he'd already tried. Yet both received their intimations of possibility from the same internal source, from which all of us should now be drawing our inspiration and hope.

Real vision comes not from what we see in the past or the future; it emerges from what we see within. The soul is the only safe repository for our dreams of a reborn world. It is the soul that will direct us—no matter what our age—to the role we can best play in realigning the earth with the consciousness of heaven. We have within us, through an internal guidance system created by God Himself, all the instructions we need in order to midwife a new world. Both our temporal and eternal selves are programmed perfectly for what we need to do now.

And I do mean now.

Dear God,
Please prepare me,
heart and soul,
to bring light into darkened times.
Amen

History moves forward one insight at a time. From the Jewish embrace of a monotheistic God to Buddha's vision of compassion; from the teaching of Jesus that God is love to Martin Luther's insistence that we can talk to Him ourselves; from the individual's creative genius spurred by the Italian Renaissance to the philosophical maturity of the European Enlightenment; from the genius of the American Experiment to the invention of quantum physics—the march of armies is creatively small compared to the march of ideas. And that is the purpose of time, for both the individual and the species: that as life progresses, our understanding can mature.

All of us take two steps forward and one step back at times, but there is nevertheless an evolutionary impulse—within every heart, every cell, and every aspect of life—marching ahead despite all resistance. Our task is to consciously conspire with that impulse, in full partnership with the force of love at the center of all things, entwined with its divine pulsation and heat, both riding and directing the wave by which humanity shall rise up at last.

IT'S AMAZING HOW MANY PEOPLE today do not take it for granted that the planet will survive the next 50 years. Whether from weather disasters or military misadventures, there are so many ways we could be destroyed.

Rationally, this is certainly true. But spiritual power is nonrational. That's not to say it's *irrational*, just nonrational. It springs forth from a quantum field not limited by mortal circumstances. The catastrophic possibilities that threaten the world today reflect who we have been until now, and they'll stay the way they are for as long as we stay the way *we* are. The possibility for a miraculous change in global affairs reflects the possibility for miraculous change in us.

We are living at a time of two parallel phenomena: one world clearly falling apart and another one struggling to be born. We're called on to be both death doulas and birth doulas, helping humanity navigate the turbulent waters between the two.

Spiritual transformation, not human manipulation, is the only level fundamentally deep enough to alter the now dangerous trajectory of human history. We can't just "fix" our way out of what's going on now. We need a miracle, which we will have only if we ourselves become miracle workers.

Miracles occur naturally in the presence of love. In our natural state, we *are* miracle workers because love is who we are. Talk about personal transformation—the journey from fear to love—is not a narcissistic exercise. It's not fuzzy thinking or soft-brained woo woo. It's the most necessary component to our re-creating human society and affecting the course of history.

The problem with the world is that we've been torn from our original nature. Torn from ourselves, we become addicts. Torn from each other, we become abusers. Torn from the earth, we become its destroyers. And that tear—a separation from our divine oneness—is not a metaphor. It is not a symbol. It is a literal, vicious, insidiously progressive disease of the human spirit. It is *force*. And it has at its command the same sophisticated level of mental operating skills as does the better part of us. It is our dark side, and underestimating its sway is naïve.

When we were children, we learned about evolution. If a species came to the point where its collective behavioral patterns were no longer well-adapted for its survival, one of two things would happen: It would evolve or it would grow extinct. The path of evolution occurs when a mutation happens: A member of the species demonstrates a more sustainable way, and enough of its other members follow.

That is where humanity is today. Our collective behavioral patterns are malfunctional. From our ways of treating the environment to our ways of treating each other, we are on an ever-escalating probable path to species extinction over the next one hundred years. The mutation today is spiritual, and the survivable way forward is that we learn to love each other. We must transition—and quickly—from a model of separation and domination to a model of unity and collaboration.

Midlife is the time when we've put away the toys of childhood and are ready to take on the task of creating a more loving world.

The miracle minded are not naïve about darkness; we don't carry around cans of pink paint and pour it over everything so we can pretend things are fine. We can't invoke the dawn if we deny that night occurred. What could possibly serve darkness more than people failing to realize its sly and insidious nature? A serious grown-up is not someone who looks away from the pain of the world; a serious grown-up is someone who sees the point of our lives as committing ourselves to healing it.

Dear God,
Please forgive us for the wounded earth,
and the needless suffering
it inflicts.
Intercede on behalf of our better selves
and repair the damage done.
Replace our fear with hope, dear God,
and turn all hate to love.
Amen

EVERY ONCE IN A WHILE, people ask me what I think I would have done with my life if I hadn't found *A Course in Miracles.* I usually mention Edina on the British TV comedy *Absolutely Fabulous.* If you haven't seen it, trust me—funny, but also scary. Like that character, some people get stuck in life, circling over and over to the same old spots because they can't find the door to another set of options. Most of us at one point or another can relate to that. All I know is that the only escape for me has been a door I cannot open by myself.

Turning 40, I woke up that morning feeling very grateful for my life. I had just published *A Return to Love*, providing me with professional options I had never dreamed would be mine. I remember being told when I turned 30, "Oh, that's the age past which 'She's young' isn't an excuse anymore." Turning 40, I didn't have any pithy platitudes to guide me, but I had an inner knowing that this decade is important.

The point is to honor the unique transitions that mark our lives as we age. If we don't choose to mark them consciously—doing the deep inner dive where we ask souls what we have learned so far, and what life is asking of us in the years ahead—life has a way of marking them for us. For me, finding myself smack dab in the middle of the AIDS crisis blew the illusions of childhood right out of my consciousness. An experience in many ways so awful was also a gift in my life: It made me grow up. It showed me human suffering up close and personal in ways that scorched my soul yet left me forever blessed.

Americans have had a prolonged post-adolescence, remaining a bit immature past the point when we should long ago have been giving up the toys of childhood. We live in a noxious pink cloud of marketing, an assault disguised as a gift to ourselves, a demonic dance seducing us to buy things that things simply cannot give. Yet even now, nature's intelligence is weighing in on that. Current events are not the stuff of child's play. Maturity is no longer requested, it's demanded. When it's time to grow up, life has a way of making sure we most probably will.

Midlife is the age when you're still young enough to do anything, yet old enough to know that you should be doing something important. Yeah, you can continue to play games with yourself and others, but you can't feel good about yourself if you do. You're looking for a life of greater meaning and respect—as you should be. That greater life is looking for you too.

Remember that song about "looking for love in all the wrong places"? Or maybe you don't, depending on your age, but the lyric still hits a nerve. The key at midlife is to look not only for love but for all forms of sustenance and meaning beyond the immature landscape of modern culture. Raising children is serious business. Showing up for your country is serious business. Saving the planet is serious business. And they are the business you were born to do.

Many years ago, I was complaining to a therapist about a book deadline I was feeling pressure to meet. At the end of the session, she said to me, "I hope time slows down for you this week." Her words stunned me. As someone involved in metaphysics, I knew that time is relative, but I had never before recognized such practical application of that knowledge to my life. It wasn't that I had to rush to meet the deadline; it's that I had to slow done enough within myself to allow myself to do it. Slowing down inside, I would achieve more in the same amount of time.

Now apply that to age. In our 40s, we feel the first physical signs of slowing down. Not anything yet that freaks us out, of course. There's nothing yet that we can't do. It's simply that we somehow start to take a more adult stride through life. Your nervous system is supporting your entrance into an inwardly more mature life.

There is a way to move into that slower, what you might call timeless realm my therapist told me about all those years ago: meditation. Whether we enter the space from a religious, spiritual, or secular place doesn't matter. What matters is that we sink into the realm beyond the mortal mind, beyond concepts and chatter, to find ourselves at home at last.

For me, connection to God means connection to a field of all-knowing. All-powerful Love from which my life is inseparable. In *A Course in Miracles*, it says, "You think you have many different problems, but you really only have one: your separation from God." In thinking we are disconnected from our Source, we disconnect from ourselves. We forget who we are. We divide into fractals of personality, our wholeness surrendered to the illusion of randomness. And that is why we suffer.

Sometimes when I wake up in the morning, I can feel my soul reach up to God, my mind uttering phrases from the Workbook of *A Course in Miracles* workbook that I keep next to my bed. I'm hardly some contemporary version of Saint Teresa—I'm just exhausted from a life of searching for anything but the be-all and end-all. My soul has been thrown against so many rocky cliffs, and I finally realized I was the wind. Who else but God could calm the tempest in my soul? And I have a feeling, having been calm for certain moments and certain hours and certain days, that what happens when I achieve that state is not just useful to me, but to those around me. Finding inner peace brings peace to all.

EVERY PROBLEM IS A CHALLENGE to become a better person. Imagine, then, what we're being challenged to become in order to turn history around right now. What quantum leap will transition us from the level of consciousness at which we created our problems to a level at which we miraculously solve them? Who is it we are destined to be, that in our presence the dense thought-forms of hate will simply drop away?

That's what is so exhilarating about this moment. Given that God has an answer to every problem the moment it occurs, then there exists in His mind an absolute plan—a blueprint for our salvation—already etched in full upon our hearts. According to that plan, we'll be individually and collectively redeemed and set upon a new path of evolution. All the old notions will die away, and the human race will remember at last that we were conceived in love; we are here to love; and one way or another, we'll remember to love.

One of the most important things that any of us can do to help the world are to pray and meditate consistently. Prayer, according to *A Course in Miracles,* is the conduit of miracles. It changes us, and through us, the entire world. No one who prays and meditates consistently doesn't give a damn what happens.

The first reason we pray and meditate is to handle the darkness of the world, strengthening our resistance to rampant chaos and negativity. In this time of historical phase transition, many people are experiencing a low-grade panic they're not even aware of. All of us should surround ourselves with a shield of light, and prayer and meditation provide it.

Interestingly, however, we don't just pray and meditate so we can handle the darkness. We do it also so we can handle the light. Our nervous systems are being infused today by light streaming down in response to humanity's prayers for help. But a nervous system unprepared for such an onrush can become overloaded. It does us little good if we succeed at calling forth miracles yet are psychologically and emotionally unprepared to receive them when they arrive. Prayer not only calls forth our good but prepares us to handle it once it comes.

As Martin Luther King, Jr., said, "[We need] a qualitative change in our souls as well as a quantitative change in our lives." Many people say we're being called by the dictates of sustainability to live materially smaller lives, and perhaps this is true. But spiritually, we're being called to live *bigger* lives, to which our resistance is at least as strong.

In *A Course in Miracles*, it says that those who have achieved the most in life have achieved a fraction of what all of us are capable of. Imagine that. And if we open the floodgates to our full potential now, do we get to retrieve whatever possibilities we failed to manifest over the previous years in our lives?

When we don't grow in certain areas, we can experience a kind of "flat line" while those around us gradually climb as in a diagonal line on a graph. Yet once we awaken to whatever awareness returns us to the natural arc of our soul growth, we make a direct vertical ascent to the place we were supposed to be—where we *would* have been had we not tarried. This often happens when people get sober;

all of a sudden, positive energy springs forth that they'd suppressed during the years they were using.

Even if you're not an addict, just by living in this society you've been privy to an addictive system.

It's time for all of us to get emotionally and psychologically sober now . . . to awaken from the stupor of the last few decades. To claim the percentage of our potential that we haven't yet manifested and go for that 100 percent. The race is on. This is it. Let's pray. Let's go.

OUR PROBLEM ISN'T THAT WE DON'T THINK love is an important thing; our problem is that we don't think it's the *most* important thing. There are lots and lots of distractions out there.

But something happens when you've seen enough. Children suffering needlessly . . . kids going off to war . . . people dying of hunger in a world of plenty; lesser issues begin to pale in comparison. Midlife is when a certain kind of serious sets in. A day comes when you look at the news and say, *What the hell are we doing?!*

It's time to stand for something; that, to me, is the meaning of midlife. We stand for ourselves and we stand for the world. Yet we also understand that there are forces among us that stand for something else. So remember, conviction is a force multiplier. With so many people in the world convicted in their hate, the only hope for the world is that a whole lot more of us will now be convicted in our love.

With every thought of love, we participate in the creation of a unified field of exponentially greater possibility for everyone. When a butterfly flaps its wings near the tip of South America, it affects the wind patterns near the North Pole. And the same is true in the realm of consciousness: Every miracle you work in your life is a blessing on life itself.

Love is to fear what light is to darkness; in the presence of one, the other disappears. When enough of us stand in the light of true love—not a simplistic love, but the strong and extraordinary love of God—then all that is not love will cease. But not until then. Until enough of us learn to love as God loves, creating a force field of holiness to purify the earth and dissolve its evil, then we're going to continue our march toward planetary disaster.

Love *is* the answer. Yet look at how terrifying that thought is to the ego. We find that notion—that love is our salvation—more frightening than war, do we not? We resist it more than we resist nuclear disaster. And why? Because the love of which I speak is one that would transcend the ego, and the world we live in is the ego's delight. The ego knows that by embracing love, we're destroying *it.* But those are our only choices, really: the fear-based ego will survive, or we will.

NOT EVERYONE HAS MONEY OR WORLDLY POWER, but all of us have equal capacity to think, intend, and pray with conviction. Love is an ever-renewable spiritual resource. We wouldn't have to worry so much about the state of the world if we felt more universal agreement among us that we'll all do whatever we can to heal it.

No matter who we are, we have things we're supposed to do to fulfill the calling of our souls. But the soul's calling isn't a broad revelation that will be written in large letters across the sky. Rather, it's a challenge to be the person we're capable of being in any given moment. We never know what conversation or encounter could lead to what, as long as we're showing up for it as best we can. God's universe is itself one big loving intention, and when you align your own intentions with His, you set in motion a spiritual wind at your back. I missed so many opportunities in my life not because they didn't arrive, but because when they did, my mind was elsewhere.

Hatred and fear don't have this cosmic support; while they have power, they don't have *spiritual* power. And they're spiritually powerless when confronted by a genuine love. There are terrible things in the news today, but as much darkness as there is out there, there is more love *in here.* Perhaps that's what the bigger problems of the world are here for, in some way: They challenge us to dig deeper into ourselves for who we really are and how we might choose to live differently. Martin Luther King, Jr., said that it's time to inject a new kind of love into the veins of human civilization. That love *is* rising up today. It's a new kind of thinking, a great turning of the heart.

In every area—from medicine to education to business to media to politics to the arts—there are people expressing new, more enlightened modes of being and behavior. And each of us, no matter who we are, can align ourselves with a better idea. A world is crumbling, but a new one is emerging. When we consciously commit to creating a more loving planet, then that which is not love will fall of its own dead weight.

When all of this comes together, the world will change in the twinkling of an eye.

Dear God,
I place the world in Your hands.
Please use me
to help make things right.
Amen

Chapter Nine

We Are the World

Particularly as we get older, our spirits as well as our bodies need more quiet time, reflection, and simple immersion in the magic of just *being*. That doesn't mean we're retreating from the world; we're moving into a deeper experience of it. For what constitutes the world is a whole lot bigger than what we see with our physical eyes. Part of the value of the aging process—and I did say that, yes: the *value* of the aging process—is that it delivers us naturally to realms in which we're not quite so tethered to the realities of the material world. It's not so much that we're losing something as that we're *finding* something. I find it liberating to have forgotten certain things; thank *God* I forgot them! And that's not to minimize scary monsters such as the fear of dementia. It's just to keep some of our changes in perspective.

I don't think as quickly as I used to, I'm sure of it. Nor do I speak as quickly or move as quickly. But it seems to me that I think more deeply. It's like I understand things in the round.

I WOKE UP ONCE TO A LATE-NIGHT EPIPHANY that shone like a neon pronouncement: that the key to human salvation lies in our living for each other. I know, I know. Hardly new. But at the moment it came to me, it seemed big and profound.

Obviously we've all heard the concept before, but aren't we stymied by what it actually means? Does it mean that we're supposed to give all of our possessions to the poor? How does that work in terms of our worldly responsibilities? Are we not supposed to have a home for our children? Aren't we supposed to provide for them? And is it bad to enjoy nice things?

In *A Course in Miracles,* it says: "To have, give all to all." But sometimes you look at the material world and think, *Well, surely it can't mean that. . . .*

The line I heard in my head that night was not "Give away everything you own." It was simply "Live for others." And I've wondered what the world would look like if we did.

We've been so thoroughly programmed to look out for number one, as though "me" is so much more important than "we." But the shift from living for ourselves to living for others is the spiritual imperative calling humanity back to the garden.

In the human body, every cell is filled with a guiding intelligence. Some cells are guided to the pancreas, others to the brain, others to the lungs, and so forth. There, they perform a collaborative function, joining with other cells to serve the healthy functioning of the organ and organism they are part of.

Sometimes, however, a cell disconnects from that natural intelligence and goes off to do its own thing. It joins with other similarly "forgetful" cells, forming their own alternative kingdom. Obviously, that's cancer. That alternative kingdom is the malignant tumor which, having forgotten to serve the organ of which it was part, now moves to invade and destroy it.

Such is what has happened to the human race. We have been infected by a malignant consciousness—the thought that it's "all about me." We see ourselves as separate competitors instead of natural collaborators. And we are literally destroying ourselves.

What, then, about healthy boundaries? Does living for others mean I'm to give everyone everything—as in my time, my energy, my money, my heart? I've tried to do that . . . be the paragon of self-sacrifice . . . never having time for myself, making myself wrong for wanting to take care of me, always running around trying to please or do for others. And it got me nowhere. If anything, it left me angry, resentful, vulnerable to thieves, and feeling much more stuck in a rut on my spiritual path as opposed to being sped up on it. Wrecked half the time, I rarely showed up as my best for anyone.

Healthy boundaries *are* loving; they show respect both to the person who sets them and to the person who's asked to honor them. I think it's best to seek a balanced life, at peace with ourselves and our own loved ones; then when we do turn our attention to the world, we can bring so much more to it. We bring a higher version of ourselves.

According to *A Course in Miracles,* sacrifice has no place in God's universe. Taking care of ourselves in a righteous way *is* meaningful service to a greater task because we cannot give what we cannot be. From that space of peace, and the moderate behavior it produces, comes more than enough money and time and energy to give to the world. Service is very serious work, but codependency it is not.

So how, then, do we live for others? I see it as a way of being. It's a generous heart. It means I can make the person who just carried my bags into the hotel room feel how much I truly appreciate what he did for me. Tip him generously as well, of course, but match the tip with an attitude of respect for what he does. Both are important. It means that in any moment, as part of my spiritual practice, I can do what I can to show love and respect for the person in front of me, on the phone with me, or whatever. Even if you get the big things right, failing at the little ones can bite you in the ass.

Most of us have more contact with other human beings each day than we might realize, and with every encounter, there's a chance for a miracle. There's the person behind the counter when you bought your coffee. The person on the phone when you made that call about getting your dryer serviced. The person who washes the windows in your office building. It might not seem like much, this tiny little droplet of compassion added to the universe when you show up more kindly, but the important point is not what it did for the universe. The point is what it did for *you*—it changed *you*—and that is how it shifts your world. All minds are joined in spirit, and the tiniest particle of compassion can have wide-ranging effects.

Throughout my childhood my father told a story that obviously he had trouble letting go. He was walking quickly down the street one day when a colleague, sitting in an outdoor space, said, "Hey Sam, sit down and have a cup of coffee with me!"

My father was rushing to the courthouse. "Can't!" he said. "I'm in a hurry."

Soon afterward, the gentleman killed himself. It was a lesson my father did not forget; his feelings of guilt clearly stayed with him for years. Every time I hear or read in an anti-suicide advertisement, "Reach out for help," I think how often someone had probably already tried that and been rebuffed. We've all been there. We never know how one small bit of compassion can make a difference in someone's life.

Holiness is a shift in purpose; the effort to live every moment conscious of our purpose as God's representatives on earth. The point of any moment is to receive love and to extend it. It's not that it's *difficult* to do, usually. What's difficult is getting over our resistance to doing it. It's a different mindset, a different kind of emotional and psychological mindset. We do spiritual practice in order to culture the musculature of a loving heart and mind, and every situation in our lives will give us a chance to practice.

Anything we do that honors only ourself is simply a spiritual dead end. There's no cosmic blessing supporting it. But anything done with others in mind—even if it involves caring for ourselves so we can be more prepared and available to serve others—is what Buddha would call right living.

Consider a vacation, for instance. It betters you to give your body and mind a rest every once in a while. A holiday increases the healthy bonds among partners, friends, and family. The principle of service doesn't require you to avoid joyous opportunities; if anything, joy is an emotional stimulant. Go for it! *A Course in Miracles* says the purpose of our lives is to be happy.

There's time for fun, and there's time for work. The relationship between the two seems to be a pattern within all natural systems; you can feel it in your gut whether you're on or off track. When your life is all fun and no work, you feel unclean somehow. When it's all work and no fun, you're out of balance and hardly of use to anyone. In fact, it's because the problems of the world *are* so serious that we need to do whatever it takes to lighten up sometimes. One of the ways you know you're in the flow is if you're simultaneously seriously of service and seriously enjoying yourself. It feels right because it *is* right. At the deepest level, our needs are all one.

A 62-YEAR-OLD FRIEND OF MINE was telling me recently that he was thinking of retiring.

"I don't see you retiring," I told him. "I think you're on the brink of discovering what you came here to do."

In the last few years we've seen an interesting trend: The "second career" has become a new buzz. People who have spent 20, 30, or 40 years achieving one thing then take up something else. What used to be seen as retirement age is now seen, if the person wishes, as simply career Phase Two. Rather than thinking of the second career as an anticlimax or "just a little something I do to stay busy," people end up seeing the first, perhaps more flashy work as a prelude to something more important that they're meant to be doing with their lives. They view achievements that were the height of their material success to have been preparation for an even greater success—the means by which they learned the skills they'd ultimately need to make their biggest contribution to the world.

The new midlife becomes a time when the *Sturm und Drang* of our more youthful years is alchemized into the highest manifestation of our talents: something useful not only to ourselves but to others. It might take 10 years to discover how to build a business and then another 10 to learn how to be the most compassionate human being—add 10 more to find out how to be the best mate or parent, and somewhere around our 50s or 60s we're ready to live our most shining lives.

From people who have hated their jobs for decades and now burst free at last to live their true calling, to those who have loved their careers but want to reach for something more meaningful in midlife or beyond, something new is happening. Closing shop is not the pulse of this moment.

A 50-year-old today might have 20, 30, or even 40 good work years left. We still have time. But this is a moment on the planet, if ever there was one, when all hands are needed on deck. And it's not just young hands, with their physical power, that are needed. Also needed are the hands of those who are guided by the wisdom only years can bring. Many of us carry within us a memory of a time when the world we live in seemed more full of hope. That hope is missing now, and our job is to restore it.

AS I WRITE THIS, it's a turbulent time in the world. For those of us in free societies, there are challenges to our freedom we never expected in our lifetimes. But our power as healers and repairers of the world rests on nothing but our commitment. As soon as we say, "God, please use me," He will. You'll be amazed at the way the universe works for you, once you go to work for the universe.

Dear God,
In these momentous times,
please use me.
Make me the person you would have me be
So I can do the things you would have me do.
In whatever way I can serve Love best
Please show me how.
Amen

We are now in the midst of a great revolution, a quantum leap from one era of human history to another. Things are going to be radically different over the next few years, as we will enter either a new age of darkness or a new age of light.

Humanity's grace period has ended now. We will fundamentally change, or we will cease to be as a species on this planet. There's a new conversation in the air today, and all of us should contribute our voices to it as best we can. It is time to redesign the world—not along traditional economic geopolitical lines, but along deeply humanitarian ones—in which the amelioration of unnecessary human suffering becomes the new organizing principle of human civilization.

I heard someone say recently, "The hippies were right about everything." I laughed loudly and said, "THANK YOU!" The mistake of the '60s generation wasn't that we didn't have the right goals. But we didn't yet realize all the means by which they're achieved. In the words of Gandhi, "The end is inherent in the means." We must *be* the change we want to see happen in the world, *because otherwise the change will not happen.* We had the right politics and dedication to love. What we didn't know yet was how to merge them. Now we do. Today we're more sophisticated about politics and more sophisticated about love. Our job is to be holistic, whole-person activists, bringing all of ourselves—our mind and our heart, our thoughts and our behavior—to the task of saving the world.

Politics and economics must mirror our spirituality or else they mock it. Humanity will change; the only issue now is whether we do so because we act wisely, or because the pain of not changing becomes so intense that nature will give us no choice. A nuclear bomb would ruin everyone's day and everyone's business. There is nothing astute—financially, or in any other way—about doing whatever we want to do without worrying about its effect on others. Such thinking must be repudiated now, in ourselves and in others. It's time to transcend modernity's separatist mindset and lay claim to a more enlightened worldview.

It's said that when Ralph Waldo Emerson visited Henry David Thoreau in jail after he was sentenced for his protests against the Mexican-American War, he asked his friend what he was doing in there—and Thoreau responded, "What are you doing *out there*?" That's how it feels to be someone shouting, "WE'VE GOT TO CHANGE!" at the top of our lungs today; anyone who isn't saying that must be nuts.

Age gives you the freedom to know what you know, own what you know, and say what you know without caring who does or does not agree. The only justification you need for having an opinion is that it's your opinion. You might be right and you might be wrong, but under no condition will you be silent about what you believe. As Jesus said in the Gospel of Thomas: "That which you have will save you if you bring it forth from yourselves. That which you have within you will kill you if you do not bring it forth."

One of the ways we give birth to a new world is by speaking it into existence. *Love* is far from a weak word: It is the power of one word, one prayer, one book, one speech, one conversation, one poem, one script, one campaign, one song at a time. If we speak of love, our word will prevail—if we flood the field, if we take the hits, if we endure the mockery, if we accept disapproval, if we endure condescension, if we grieve but accept the lack of support from those who know better yet turn away when we do. It is part of the journey to face the fires of fierce resistance to the ways of love. The world is in the midst of a spiritual battle, though the ego fights and love does not fight back. It simply is, spoken and expressed until we reach that critical mass.

"MINE EYES HAVE SEEN THE GLORY of the coming of the Lord: / He is trampling out the vintage where the grapes of wrath are stored; / He hath loosed the fateful lightning of His terrible swift sword: / His truth is marching on."

We watched Judy Garland sing those lyrics to "The Battle Hymn of the Republic" on television after the assassination of President Kennedy. I was too young to appreciate the full import of what was happening, but my parents' tears and Judy Garland's performance have stayed with me forever. A mental snapshot of Garland singing that song has stayed in my head for over 40 years. Its message is still one of my favorite affirmations that no matter what happens, no matter how much cruelty or injustice fills the world, God's truth will somehow prevail.

In order to "[trample] out the vintage where the grapes of wrath are stored" (cancel out hate) and "[loose] the fateful lightning of His terrible swift sword" (*karma* and *justice* are gentler words, but you don't edit Julia Ward Howe), God needs our help as much as we need His. She ended the song with these words: "As He died to make men holy, let us live to make men free." If only.

THEN, OF COURSE, AT THE END OF ALL THIS—after all the years of yearning and strife, both achievement and disappointment—we will lay down the body. All of us hope for that tunnel of light, the otherworldly peace we've read about, and the joy of feeling that in the final analysis, this lifetime wasn't all that bad.

Death can be seen as our next adventure. In the words of Carl Jung, "Shrinking away from death is something unhealthy and abnormal which robs the second half of life of its purpose." That doesn't mean death is something to be excited about. But it's something to be accepted in faith—faith that nothing exists outside the love of God, the perfection of God, or the plan of God. The body is but a suit of clothes, to be treated as the precious gift it is until such time when the spirit no longer has need of it. At the point when we're to leave here, it's by definition into greater Light.

Knowing that we will die doesn't make life less important; in fact, it makes it more so. The realization of our mortality creates a sense of urgency to use life wisely, to appreciate it fully, to love more deeply while we're still here and we still can. There is a magical thinking to youth: We often have the secret thought that we're the one who's going to cheat death. And with that false sense that life lasts forever can come a casual disregard for how serious it is. I now see that when I was young, the things I took most seriously were mainly unimportant things. It's only with age that we came to see how important, how deeply important, is the simple existence of life itself.

When you're young it never occurs to you that when you call a friend, it's not one of an endless number of times you'll have the chance to do that. Once you viscerally appreciate that every experience in the material world is finite, you realize how amazing it is just to be able to make that call. Any thing we do could be the last time we do it.

When we're young, we don't know, except intellectually, that we won't always have endless energy or glow. When age forces us to see how much is gone, we're shocked and hurt to realize all the things that are over and will not come again.

But then something happens when the shock wears off . . . something subtle yet immense. What happens is counter to the thinking of the world. We'd always seen older people when we were out in the world, and we looked down on their diminished lives with pity. What we failed to realize—how could we then?—was that many of them were looking at *us* as the pitiable ones. For we did not yet realize what life was about or even really for. They were having, perhaps, more fun than we knew. They were seeing, surely, what we had not yet seen. What happens in time is that we enter their room. It isn't what we had expected. It's whatever we *want* it to be. . . .

Dear God,
As I age,
make me ever more
the person You would have me be.
For I would know the joy of life
before my days are done.
Amen

I INTERVIEWED A WOMAN on my radio show who'd had lupus for two decades; had been married to a man for many years who told her on Christmas Eve, while she was wrapping her small children's presents, that he didn't want to be married anymore; had lost one of her children suddenly in a violent accident; and is now married to a practicing alcoholic. I felt such admiration for her that she simply wakes up each morning to face another day. Any one of those things might have knocked me out for years.

I don't know what it is that keeps us coming back up. When I think of what people have experienced—from Auschwitz to Rwanda to Iraq to everyday Americans just trying to survive—I can hardly stand it. Sometimes I think that the oceans are a material manifestation of humanity's tears. Clearly there is some tenacity, some deeper longing to keep keeping on, that lies at the heart of the human experience. I don't think we cleave to life for no other reason than that we're afraid of death. I think we cleave to life out of a deeper knowing that there is something about it, something profoundly beautiful, that simply hasn't happened yet.

Like salmon rushing upstream, we instinctively know we're here to continue the process of life. That we *are* the process of life. We're here to contribute to a larger drama than our individual selves could ever fathom, much less describe.

At the end of Stanley Kubrick's movie masterpiece *2001: A Space Odyssey,* an infant is seen floating through outer space. Surely that's the ultimate goal: the birth of a new humanity. Yet if that child is to be born, we all need to parent it. Conceived in our minds and hearts, it will be fed by our compassionate action. This new delightful and delighted being is gestating within us all. Wars and rumors of war abound, that is true. But people continue to fall in love. People continue to atone for their mistakes. People continue to forgive and to ask for forgiveness. And people continue to hope and pray. The point, when staring death in the face, is to proclaim more life. And we are doing that.

I believe in a compassionate God. It takes only one moment's epiphany, one moment's prayer, one moment's genuine and humble desire to do right by love to invoke His intervention in the irresponsible drama of a reckless humanity. As we look not back or forward, but deep within, we see a light that is greater than the darkness of the world. It's a hope that surpasses the understanding of the world, and a love that is greater than the hatred in the world.

Seeing that light, we must follow that light through the birth canal toward humanity's rebirth. While our labor is long and in many ways hard, we are being born to something huge and precious. We are being born to our own true selves. And we will never settle, ever again, for being less than we truly are.

Dear God,
May love prevail
in us and in the world.
May our aging
Only improve our understanding,
Deepen our wisdom,
And increase our joy.
Then, dear God,
Help us bring the gifts
You have given us
As our gifts
To all the world
Amen

Acknowledgments

Thank you so much to the team at Hay House for allowing me to bring this book to new life. I'm grateful to my friends Reid Tracy and Patty Gift for approving the project. Editor Anne Barthel was a marvelous guide and editorial companion throughout the process.

Many people come together to bring a book into the world. I'm also grateful to Tricia Breidenthal, Julie Davison, and Kirsten Callais for design, Monica O'Connor for editorial assistance, Celeste Johnson for production and editorial management, and Steve Morris for managing the audio production.

Thanks to Lauren Selsky, Tammy Vogsland, and Ellis Levine for keeping my world afloat as I wrote this.

My deepest appreciation to all of you. It's an honor to be on the team.

About the Author

For more than four decades, Marianne Williamson has been a leader of spiritually progressive circles. She is the author of 16 books, four of which have been #1 *New York Times* bestsellers. A quote from the mega-bestseller *A Return to Love,* "Our deepest fear is not that we are inadequate. Our deepest fear is that we are powerful beyond measure . . . " is considered an anthem for a contemporary generation of seekers.

Her other bestsellers have included *A Woman's Worth, The Law of Divine Compensation, Tears to Triumph, The Gift of Change, Everyday Grace,* and *The Mystic Jesus: The Mind of Love.* With her books and online classes, she has taught millions of people universal spiritual themes at the heart of all the great religions of the world.

Williamson founded Project Angel Food, a non-profit organization that has delivered more than 19 million meals to ill and dying homebound patients in the Los Angeles area since 1989. The group was created to help people suffering from the ravages of HIV/AIDS. She has also worked throughout her career on poverty, anti-hunger, and racial reconciliation issues. In 2004, she co-founded The Peace Alliance and supported the creation of a U.S. Department of Peace.

She ran for the Democratic nomination for President in both 2020 and 2024.

Instagram: **@MarianneWilliamson**
Website: **Marianne.com**
Substack: **MarianneWilliamson.Substack.com**
YouTube: **https://www.youtube.com/@MarianneWilliamsonCommunity**

Notes

Notes

Notes

NOTES

Notes

Hay House Titles of Related Interest

YOU CAN HEAL YOUR LIFE, the movie,
starring Louise Hay & Friends
(available as an online streaming video)
www.hayhouse.com/louise-movie

THE SHIFT, the movie,
starring Dr. Wayne W. Dyer
(available as an online streaming video)
www.hayhouse.com/the-shift-movie

•••••••

THE AWAKENED WAY: Making the Shift to a Divinely Guided Life by Suzanne Giesemann

HIGHER PURPOSE: How to Find More Inspiration, Meaning, and Purpose in Your Life by Robert Holden

SOVEREIGN: Reclaim Your Freedom, Energy, and Power in a Time of Distraction, Uncertainty, and Chaos by Emma Seppälä, Ph.D.

THE UNIVERSE HAS YOUR BACK: Transform Fear to Faith by Gabrielle Bernstein

WELL BEING: A Story of Healing from Autoimmune Disease and a Guide to Charting Your Own Path to Wellness by Valentina Gaylord

YOU'RE IN THE RIGHT PLACE: Let Go of the Past, Make Friends with Uncertainty, and Discover the Magic of an Uncharted Future by Colette Baron-Reid

•••••••

We hope you enjoyed this Hay House book. If you'd like to receive our online catalog featuring additional information on Hay House books and products, or if you'd like to find out more about the Hay Foundation, please contact:

HAY HOUSE

Hay House LLC, P.O. Box 5100, Carlsbad, CA 92018-5100
(760) 431-7695 or (800) 654-5126
www.hayhouse.com® • www.hayfoundation.org

Published in Australia by:
Hay House Australia Publishing Pty Ltd
18/36 Ralph St., Alexandria NSW 2015
Phone: +61 (02) 9669 4299
www.hayhouse.com.au

Published in the United Kingdom by:
Hay House UK Ltd
1st Floor, Crawford Corner,
91–93 Baker Street, London W1U 6QQ
Phone: +44 (0)20 3927 7290
www.hayhouse.co.uk

Published in India by:
Hay House Publishers (India) Pvt Ltd
Muskaan Complex, Plot No. 3,
B-2, Vasant Kunj, New Delhi 110 070
Phone: +91 11 41761620
www.hayhouse.co.in
